Health Promotion and Professional Ethics

by
Alan Cribb and Peter Duncan

Blackwell
Science

© 2002 by Blackwell Science Ltd,
a Blackwell Publishing Company
Editorial Offices:
Osney Mead, Oxford OX2 0EL, UK
   Tel: +44 (0)1865 206206
Blackwell Science Inc., 350 Main Street,
Malden, MA 02148-5018, USA
   Tel: +1 781 388 8250
Iowa State Press, a Blackwell Publishing
Company, 2121 State Avenue, Ames, Iowa
50014-8300, USA
   Tel: +1 515 292 0140
Blackwell Science Asia Pty, 54 University Street,
Carlton, Victoria 3053, Australia
   Tel: +61 (0)3 9347 0300
Blackwell Wissenschafts Verlag,
Kurfürstendamm 57, 10707 Berlin, Germany
   Tel: +49 (0)30 32 79 060

First published 2002 by Blackwell Science Ltd

Library of Congress
Cataloging-in-Publication Data
Cribb, Alan.
   Health promotion and professional ethics/by
   Alan Cribb and Peter Duncan.
      p. cm.
   Includes bibliographical references and index.
   ISBN 0-632-05603-7 (alk. paper)
   1. Health promotion – Moral and ethical
   aspects.   2. Medical ethics.   I. Duncan, Peter.
   II. Title.
   RA427.8 .C75 2001
   174′.2 – dc21   2001043512

ISBN 0-632-05603-7

A catalogue record for this title is available from the
British Library

Set in 10 on 13pt Times
by DP Photosetting, Aylesbury, Bucks
Printed and bound in Great Britain by
TJ International, Padstow, Cornwall

For further information on
Blackwell Science, visit our website:
www.blackwell-science.com

Health Promotion and
Professional Ethics

Contents

Preface

The primary audience for this book is health professionals on pre-service or in-service education programmes. These days health professionals and would-be professionals are required to have thought about, and take an active interest in, a wide range of issues which extend far beyond clinical knowledge and skills. As a result both health promotion and ethics have become common currency in health professional education, and there are a number of accessible introductions available to both of these fields. A further text, which links the two fields, requires some justification.

Perhaps we should first stress what this book is not meant to be. It is not a more specialised or esoteric discussion which focuses on some relatively obscure overlap between health promotion and ethics. It is first and foremost designed to be accessible and to introduce the reader to both fields of study. The two fields are linked together in the book simply because, we argue, the two fields are linked together in practice. And this linkage, we suggest, is far from obscure but something quite basic and of widespread relevance. This argument is what we hope makes the book original, and hence worth producing and reading. The full argument for the linkage is set out in the text (particularly the first two chapters) – but it can also be signalled here. The point is that as health workers bring the idea of 'promoting health' within their remit they thereby re-orient the ends, the means, and the dilemmas associated with their work. To take up health promotion is, in part, to take up a 'new professional ethics'.

We have deliberately chosen the label 'professional ethics' for our theme rather than a label such as 'bioethics', and it is worth briefly setting out why. By 'professional ethics' we mean to refer to the routine, day-to-day, value judgements inherent in, or deliberately made within, professional activity. To think about professional ethics, in this sense, requires us to be self-conscious about the values built into policies and practices, the different ways in which our choices and actions impact upon others, the standards of conduct expected from people working in our occupational field, and the need to be able to explain and defend our practice to managers and clients. None of this is an abstract, academic or theoretical activity – it is, as we say, routine stuff. Nevertheless it is necessary to stress this foundation here because (as will be discussed more fully later) there is no established 'professional ethics' in the field of health promotion.

We have also shied away from the label 'bioethics' because much of the book is not about bioethics in the widely accepted sense of moral philosophy about health care. Bioethics or health care ethics is a hugely important tradition of academic work which provides both an analytical and a critical perspective on professional ethics. We cannot pretend to do this tradition of work justice in this context but we have included it as one of the threads in our discussion, and have hopefully provided some pointers to those who feel the need to go beyond the 'common sense' of professional ethics to a more philosophically reflective stance on health care ethics. A feature of this emphasis on professional ethics rather than bioethics is our choice of deliberately mundane and non-dramatic examples of health promotion work. Whereas moral philosophy texts often embrace 'science fiction' examples or life and death dramas we have chosen to explore some of the issues through 'bread and butter' cases. Our choice here is certainly not meant to imply that the more dramatic examples are not valuable or practically important; it is merely to highlight the pervasiveness of value judgements in occupational practice.

Hopefully the organisation of the book is straightforward. The three sections each have a different role which is explained by their titles – *Why health promotion ethics?; Values and ethics in health promotion practice*; and *Towards ethically defensible health promotion*. The first and last sections serve respectively to introduce and 'take forward' the issues. Their job is adequately summarised by the synopsis contained in this Preface. The middle section has broadly the same aspirations but seeks to address these through a more careful and concrete consideration of issues in practice. We have added an introduction to Section Two to explain and illustrate this further.

We will be delighted if readers leave the text with a heightened sense of the need for a revised approach to professional ethics in an era of health promotion. But we also hope that they will be persuaded of the value of more theoretical and critical reflection on both health promotion and ethics.

Section One
Why Health Promotion Ethics?

Chapter 1
Values and Health Promotion:
Some Fundamentals

Premise and purpose

The premise of this book is that health promotion represents a challenge to the values and ethics of health professionals. The purpose of the book is to illustrate the nature of this challenge in practical terms and, we hope, to help meet it. Section One – this chapter and the following one – form an introduction to these issues and to the rest of the book. At this stage we might be expected to run into a series of definitions and clarifications: 'What is health promotion? What, for that matter, is health? What do we mean by "the values and ethics of health professionals"?' All of these questions are important and we will consider them, but we prefer to begin by approaching things indirectly.

For now we will rely on the fact that everyone reading this book must already have a notion of what is meant by health promotion. Presumably very few people would buy or borrow a book on health promotion if the term meant nothing to them! At the very least, it might be expected that you associate the term with certain kinds of activities (perhaps, for example, smoking cessation programmes). Different people may associate it with a rather different range of activities but presumably it has some such associations for everyone.

Broadening perspectives on health care

Arguably, the rise of health promotion is best understood as both a reflection and an expression of changing perspectives in health care. These changes can be seen, for example, in the broadening of curricula for the education and training of health care professionals (English National Board 1987, General Medical Council 1993). Students training to be health professionals are likely to be introduced to a wide range of disciplines, themes and topics. In addition to biological and clinical knowledge and 'hands-on' skills, they might also cover issues in psychology and sociology, aspects of law and public policy, and topics in communication as well as in ethics and in health promotion. This broadening of curricula is no doubt partly inspired by a conviction that health professionals

3

should have a broad education for their own personal and professional development; but it is mainly a consequence of evolving ideas about health and health care. Three linked trends are discernible: first, an increasing emphasis on client-centred or person-centred health care; second, an increasing emphasis on the social and environmental determinants of health; and third an increasing emphasis upon broader and more flexible notions of health and well-being.

This list of trends is clearly something of a generalisation and simplification, but in broad terms we believe it to be a reasonable summary. The trends are all elements of a reaction to what is often called, perhaps unfairly, the 'medical model'. Respectively they each provide a counterbalance to a comparatively narrow focus on 'professional authority and judgement': the nature of 'the diseased body'; and 'measures of morbidity and mortality'. In turn these health care trends are themselves a reflection of a much wider and deeper set of social trends. Although it is not within the scope of this book directly to examine these in historical or sociological detail, we can briefly remark on them. First, professional authority – and in particular professional medical authority – has been subject to fundamental critique and scepticism in many spheres. (See, for just one example, Illich 1977.) This has resulted in it being increasingly subject to influence and control from both 'below' (e.g. consumer pressures) and above (e.g. managerial pressures). Second, social and environmental sciences have increased our understanding and self-consciousness about the things which shape our lives. As a result we are likely to be more cautious about the scope for professional work alone to produce substantial changes. Third, in modern societies there is a scepticism about generalised criteria of professional success. A high priority has come to be attached to people themselves deciding what they want out of life, and what they see as contributing to their own well-being, rather than professionals attempting to decide for them.

To say that there is an increasing emphasis on these broader perspectives on health is not to suggest that they have replaced the narrower focus – merely that in many areas these counterbalances have been growing. It is arguable that there are many aspects of health care where a narrow focus still largely predominates. Furthermore, it may seem that certain important currents in health policy (e.g. evidence-based health care) amount in some respects, to a reinforcement of these narrower models. But in general, the counterbalancing trends we have identified are significant; and it is possible to see the growth of health promotion as one important reflection and expression of them.

Perhaps the fundamental point to note is that health care and the values associated with it evolve and change over time. The changing institutions and practices of health care not only represent changes in procedures and techniques; they also represent changes in values. Let us briefly consider an example – the case of the hospice movement.

Hospices are institutions which serve specific functions; i.e. providing good quality respite and terminal care for families affected by life-threatening chronic diseases. Simply to express their role in these stark terms, though, is to miss out such a lot about them. What hospices stand for, first and foremost, is a set of values. They are one answer to the question, 'How can patients and families facing life-threatening diseases, or living through the process of dying, be cared for in a way that meets their needs, respects their dignity and wishes, and does justice to all of the different forms of pain and disruption these experiences entail?'. In short, they are one institutional expression of the attempt to give 'care' a place of equal importance to 'cure' within health services. Models of good palliative care have now spread far beyond hospices themselves – indeed, many people would argue that palliative care may often be better provided for outside of specialist institutions. In many ways the legacy of hospices to health care lies in the values they represent rather than their institutional form. They are one example of the evolution of values in health care, and they highlight the tensions between 'care' and 'cure'.

The rise of the hospice movement also connects with the three trends we have just mentioned. Good palliative care aims to be centred on the patient's agenda and not that of the health professionals: it is mindful of the patient's social and cultural context, and it considers dimensions of the quality of life much broader than those defined by clinical medicine. Hospices and palliative care are of course, not just abstract 'value movements'. They also involve people undertaking different sorts of work, delivering new practices and interventions – whether it is new techniques of pharmacological pain relief, 'talking therapy', complementary approaches to health care, peer support, or many other initiatives. It is important to see that these various new practices and interventions can be subject to ethical scrutiny. We might ask, for example, about the extent to which life ought to be prolonged if it is a life which has ceased to be valued by its owner; or connected to this we might ask about how and when it is appropriate for family members to give proxy consent to the withdrawal of life sustaining treatment. Just because hospice care is performed in the name of certain 'values' it does not mean it is immune to criticism or critical examination. It is quite common for human beings to reform institutions and practices with the aim of putting an end to one set of 'evils', merely to replace them with an alternative set.

In short, health care is evolving and there are certain 'broadening' trends discernible in this evolution. We suggest that health promotion needs to be seen in this context. It connects with a set of value changes in society and is part of a range of challenges to the values of health professionals. It is also – just like the hospice movement – associated with a set of practices and interventions which again, can and should be subject to ethical scrutiny in their own right.

In the rest of this chapter, we will concentrate on exploring some of the ambiguities surrounding the idea of health promotion. This exploration involves, among other things, considering some concepts and meanings, but this concern with language is not an end in itself. In order to investigate values and ethics in health care it is essential to think about the ways in which health care is understood – at a conceptual as well as a practical level. As we have seen, changes in values represent themselves in changes in the ways things are talked about. Part of the spirit of the hospice movement, as we have mentioned, is represented by talking about the importance of 'care' and not simply 'cure'. Connected with this emphasis on care are a lot of other ideas, such as 'respect', 'compassion' or 'holism'. These can be used to develop and complement the central idea of 'care'. Similarly, the changes in perspectives and the health policy trends embodied in the health promotion movement can only be explored by looking at the ideas associated with health promotion. Unless we have a relatively clear picture of what a supporter of health promotion is actually advocating, we cannot begin to evaluate it ethically; nor are we in a position to decide whether or not a particular intervention qualifies as health promotion at all, let alone 'good' health promotion.

A tricky question: What is health promotion?

Let us now turn to the business of describing the nature of health promotion and to discussing some of the difficulties involved in doing this. The starting point for this discussion is to accept that there is no single, clear and uncontroversial account of what is meant by 'health promotion'. The term has caused, and continues to cause, considerable uncertainty and debate. (The literature of this debate is very broad, but a sense of its contentiousness can be found in Seedhouse (1997).) There are a number of approaches we could take to try and make progress in understanding: 'conceptual approaches'; 'empirical approaches'; and a combination of the two.

By a 'conceptual approach', we mean one which analyses the expression 'health promotion' and in doing so attempts to map out some coherent and circumscribed account of the meaning of the expression. Ideally, such an approach would enable us to identify some 'core sense' of the term and would help us decide to what actual processes or activities it properly applies. More realistically we would probably find that there is not simply one sense of the term, but that it can be used in rather different ways. Nevertheless, this would still help us to circumscribe the several 'core senses' of health promotion.

By an 'empirical approach', we mean one which concentrates on exploring the practices themselves (processes or activities) that people happen to call 'health promotion'. What sorts of things do people refer to as health promotion? When is the term used?

In practice, some combination of these approaches will probably be needed. This is because, on the one hand, it would seem bizarre to suppose that the 'real' (conceptual) meaning of the term was completely different from the way it was used in practice. On the other hand, if we only look at the ways in which the term is used in practice it might reveal such a variety of contradictory and confusing examples that we are left with no sense of how to 'pin down' what is meant by 'health promotion'.

We will begin by exploring a conceptual approach to answering the question. This might seem a rather abstract place to start and, as we will soon see, it is fraught with the danger of getting bogged down with rather vague-sounding concerns and debates. But despite these disadvantages, it may help us make a little progress. A purely conceptual approach might go something like this:

> *Health promotion is, by definition, the promotion of health. To promote some-thing is to encourage or increase it, so anything which encourages or increases health must be an example of health promotion. Health has a number of meanings (let us leave these on one side for now) but given any one of these meanings we are able to gain a picture of health promotion. For example, if we take health to be something like 'the absence of disease', then health promotion refers to anything which works to reduce the amount of disease in the world.*

This obviously still leaves the need for some further basic clarification. Should we think of health promotion as referring only to activities (which here we understand as things that are deliberately done); or to both activities and pro-cesses (by which we mean things that might happen without deliberate action)? Just to explore this point, take an absurd example. Suppose some freak astro-nomical event happened next year which somehow had the effect of wiping out malaria (just as an asteroid might have wiped out the dinosaurs). Would this be an example of health promotion? Or are we inclined to think that health pro-motion is something that people have 'to do', not just something which happens? For the purposes of this particular exercise let us confine health promotion to activities only.

Now there is a further piece of clarification needed. We must ask about the intention of activities. If we say health promotion refers to a set of activities: then as well as being deliberately done, must these activities be conducted with the deliberate aim of promoting health; or is what matters that an activity has the consequence of promoting health? Of course, something can be done deliberately and have consequences other than intended. Indeed, in relation to this discussion, we can imagine four kinds of activities:

(i)   activities which have the aim of promoting health and do in fact promote health;

(ii) activities which do not have the aim of promoting health but actually do promote health;

(iii) activities which have the aim of promoting health but do not promote health, and

(iv) activities which do not have the aim of promoting health and do not pro-mote health.

It seems reasonably clear that health promotion does not refer to group (iv); and that group (i) activities are good candidates for the health promotion label, but what about group (ii) and (iii) activities? If we stress the importance of the activities' *aim* then (i) and (iii) become the salient set. If we stress the importance of the activities' *consequences* then (i) and (ii) are salient.

One of the difficulties in exploring examples to illustrate these points is that there are so many other confounding factors. Not only do we have different intuitions about what counts as health, but we have different intuitions about the likely effects of different activities. Furthermore the effects of activities are typically complex. The same activity may promote health in some respects, or to some degree, whilst failing to promote health in other respects or to a different degree. These kinds of complications will become important in the detailed discussions we have about activity in Section Two. For the moment, we can use a couple of examples to explore the relevance of the broad distinction between an activity having as its *aim* the promotion of health; and an activity having this as its *consequence*. These examples will help us to recognise that this issue contains still further complications.

(1)   Suppose you are lucky enough to be able to find a plumber to install new plumbing in a house you are having modernised. She arrives one Monday morning and by Friday evening she has put in a new toilet system, a central heating system and hot and cold running water. Imagine that she spends a whole year doing this in different properties (perhaps she has a contract with a local authority or housing association to modernise its stock). It is quite possible that this activity would contribute to disease reduction and therefore (according to a model where health is understood as the absence of disease) it would be an example of health promotion. We are using it as an example of group (ii) activities above because we are supposing that the plumber does not have the aim of promoting health, and certainly does not think of what she has been doing as 'health promotion'. She sees herself as attempting to install the right equipment in technically (and perhaps aesthetically) the best way, as earning a living, as developing her competence and craft, but not as promoting health.

(2)   Suppose a hospital employee becomes privately convinced that his own 'medicinal concoction' has strong and far-reaching curative powers. As a result, he decides to add his concoction regularly (but secretly) to the hospital food whilst it is under preparation. His intention, let us imagine, is pure. He does not wish to make money or become famous. He simply wishes to make his contribution to improving the health of the hospital's patients. Unfortunately, as a consequence of this activity several patients take a serious turn for the worse having been effectively poisoned by a substance that was meant to help. This is an example of group (iii) activities. The intention is to promote health but the consequence is rather different.

Now which, if either, of these two examples should be called health promotion? To many people it will seem odd to apply the term to either. The plumbing may happen to promote health in some sense but it is not health promotion. The hospital employee may want to promote health but he is not practising health promotion. (Furthermore many people would say the same thing even if the concoction had achieved the desired effect.) Why do we suggest this? One of the reasons is that many people think of health promotion as more than the name for an abstract set of activities. They see it as the name of a specific kind of practice, like marketing or nursing. Of course, we could run into similar difficulties to those discussed above in trying to identify whether a very specific activity counted as an example of marketing or nursing – but we know in broad terms what these practices are. In following this line of thought we are, to some extent, starting to incorporate what we earlier called the 'empirical approach' – that is to say, we are reflecting on how the term 'health promotion' is used in practice.

If we think of health promotion as an occupation, like marketing or nursing, we can perhaps dismiss the above two examples fairly easily. Neither of the two protagonists has the occupation of health promotion. What is more if health promotion, like nursing, has certain conventions and standards built into it, then the hospital employee is falling short of these standards in any case. Imagine that the employee in the example is a nurse. Would we describe their activity of supplementing the food as nursing? We think not. Of course, it would be different if they were asked to do something similar as a deliberate and open feature of hospital food policy.

Now we can extend this way of thinking to health promotion. If we think of health promotion as a kind of occupational practice, then we need not get bogged down by vague hypothetical puzzles about whether or not specific isolated activities count as health promotion. Instead we need to map out the sphere of the occupational practice. We need to ask '*Who are the people who work in health promotion, and what, broadly speaking, do they do?*' So it will be possible to identify the things falling within this sphere, by virtue of being part of the occupational practice, as health promotion. (Suggesting this does not, of course, exclude the possibility of disagreements about what is 'authentic' or 'worthwhile' health promotion activity between those engaged in the overall occupational practice. Even though both sides in such disputes may argue about the specific worth of an activity being undertaken by 'the other side', they may nevertheless agree that both activities could be called 'health promotion'; their disagreement may be evaluative rather than descriptive.)

According to our first, conceptual, approach to the question, 'What is health promotion?', the answer is that it is equated, somewhat abstractly, with 'the promotion of health'. According to our second, empirical approach, health promotion is equated with a domain of occupational practice. This second approach is certainly not purely hypothetical; there are people who work in the field of health promotion and think of it as an occupation – or part of their occupation. Some of these people have health promotion in their title, and more still have the expression in their job description. The biggest group of workers unambiguously working in the field of health promotion are those whose full-time occupation is the promotion of health. Such people often (but not always) work in health promotion units attached to the health service or local authorities. In this book we will refer to these individuals as 'health promotion specialists'. Other workers who have health promotion in their job description, or who are otherwise thought of by their occupational group as practising health promotion as a significant part of their occupational role, we will refer to by the generic label 'health promoters'. A by no means exhaustive list of such workers would include nurses, midwives, health visitors, environmental health officers, teachers and doctors. (When we wish to differentiate these two groups we will use both labels; but a lot of the time we will simply use 'health promoters' to include both. There are of course many others on a possible list of occupational groups concerned with health promotion.) If we look at what is done within the occupational domain referred to as health promotion (work done by health promotion specialists and health promoters and described as health promotion), we will get a practical picture of health promotion. It includes, among other things, such activities as public health campaigns, face-to-face health education, community development work, health-related policy lobbying and planning. These are all planned activities intended to contribute to the health of groups of individuals or wider populations. But it is important to emphasise that they are a set of activities defined by their place in occupational practices and not merely the total set of activities that happen to promote health.

By and large the focus of this book will be upon health promotion as the name for the occupational practices of health promoters. We will consider the value questions faced by these groups of workers through some indicative examples. To some extent we will deliberately leave behind the conceptual issues raised in defining health promotion by taking the pragmatic solution of equating health promotion with the work most typically *called* health promotion in this field of occupations (the occupations of health promoters and health promotion specialists). This is a practical solution for what we intend to be a practical book.

Health promotion: open field or occupational field?

However, if we want to understand the nature of health promotion, it is important not to abandon the conceptual approach entirely. Part of the influence of the health promotion movement has been precisely to direct our attention to *all* the determinants of health. This is why it is properly included in, and arguably exemplifies, what we have called broadening perspectives on health care. One of the functions of the language of health promotion is to direct our attention beyond narrow health care services, and towards the myriad sets of causes and choices which shape people's experiences of health and illness. In this sense health promotion refers to an 'open field' and not merely to a set of practices and activities undertaken by occupational groups within health care and related fields alone. All activities and social and environmental processes may contribute towards the promotion of health (World Health Organisation 1986). None of them can be easily omitted from consideration.

It is for this reason that the purview of health promotion encompasses so much including: every kind of public policy – such as economic, legal, housing, transport and so on; the activities of private companies and voluntary organisations; global issues about environmental change, population growth, international capitalism; local issues about, for example, road safety or social isolation; the work and side-effects of all professional and occupational groups, and all leisure activities; and the material construction, organisation and policies of specific settings like schools and hospitals. Indeed, it encompasses just about anything you can think of! Given that all of these – and more – can have an impact on peoples' health status and experiences: and that it is therefore possible, in principle, that any of them should be taken into account as we attempt to shape and improve health; then they become worthy of the interest and attention of 'health promotion'.

Health promotion, therefore, cannot be owned by any single occupational or professional group. Anyone and everyone could be charged with some responsibility for promoting health. On the other hand there are relatively few people who would see health promotion as comprising all – or almost all – of their job description. These workers – health promotion specialists, according to our distinction – have to take into account the open field of health determinants, and consequently have to think in terms of partnerships with other individuals, organisations and sectors. However, they will also think of themselves as working at the centre of the occupational field of health promotion (other occupational fields such as nursing and medicine 'overlap' with the occupational field of health promotion) (Society of Health Education and Health Promotion Specialists 1997a).

It is characteristic of health promotion that it possesses this duality of being both a part of health care work and at the same time transcending it. Health promotion is seen as something which extends beyond, complements and perhaps even critiques, traditional health care; yet at the same time health promoters are often working in, or are closely allied to, existing health services. Indeed, as we will explore further in a later section, health promotion is increasingly seen by many as a current within health care, and as an important part of well-established health professional roles in medicine and nursing. Here again we can see the elasticity of the meaning of the term 'health promotion'. It is applied to a wide range of, sometimes contradictory, things. One of its uses seems to be simply to refer to work aimed at health which transcends narrow models of health care, even though there are some very different kinds of work which fall into this category. There is, for example, work aimed at ameliorating the environmental causes of cancer; and work aimed at improving the quality of life of cancer patients. These may both be referred to as examples of health promotion. Among the few things they have in common is that they complement – but are distinctively different from – a narrow picture of health care which concentrates on the cure of disease. In many other respects they are not at all similar to each other. Does it make sense to call them both health promotion? And, if health promotion is connected with 'the promotion of health', why should therapeutic services not be included? Before we can answer these questions we need to go down some further conceptual alleys. We need to say a little more about what counts as 'health'.

Promoting what?

We certainly do not want to get bogged down with the question, 'What is health?'; but it is not one we can completely ignore in a discussion of health promotion. It is essential to ask – both in general, and in particular cases – what exactly is being promoted in the name of health? No-one could be taken seriously if they claimed to be engaged in health promotion but were completely unable to give an account of what they thought they were promoting. Such a person would, in a basic sense, be incapable of accountability – they would not be able to give an account of what they were doing.

A lot of the elasticity in the term 'health promotion' is as a result of the elasticity in the term 'health'. There are, as we have mentioned, relatively narrow models of health and relatively broad models. There are models which are essentially 'negative': that is to say, they define health by what it is not; and models which are more positive. Representing these dichotomies are, on the one hand, the narrow and negative definition which, roughly speaking, equates health with the absence of disease; and on the other, the positive definition such as that famously produced by the World Health Organisation (WHO) in 1946:

'Health is not merely the absence of disease, but a state of complete physical, emotional, social and spiritual well-being...' (World Health Organisation 1946).

These definitions can of course be modified and clarified further. We might, for example, expand or explain 'disease' in the narrow definition to include the whole range of clinically defined deficits (including disabilities) deemed to impair health. Again by way of example, we may also wish to adapt a broader definition such as that of the WHO so it uses other words for the dimensions of well-being. Leaving these issues on one side for now, we can see that these two sorts of definition – narrow and broad – and the different models of health they represent give us very different pictures of health promotion:

(1) From the negative model and the narrow definition, health promotion is disease prevention

(2) From the positive model and the broad definition, health promotion is well-being promotion

In the contrast between these two pictures of health promotion lie many of the fundamental debates and conflicts haunting the field. The two pictures point to two very different orientations. They include different aims, will inevitably entail different approaches and will, therefore, have very different criteria of success. (Of course the two may be combined to some extent and to many people – though not everyone – (2) will seem to include (1).)

Disease prevention activities will include things like screening and vaccination. They will also include health education work and interventions attempting environmental change – if the focus of this work and these interventions is the prevention of disease. All these are, ideally, based upon epidemiological and social scientific knowledge about the causes of disease and the most effective means of intervening in those causal processes. In many ways they can be thought of as an extension of the medical approach to disease management into the social sphere. The essential difference between disease prevention-focused health promotion and therapeutic services is simply that the locus of intervention is earlier in the causal chain. The aim is to manage – and to attempt to control – the onset of disease and not merely its effects (that is to say, morbidity). Although the boundaries of 'disease prevention' are by no means clear-cut (the plumbing example applies here after all) the ends are relatively straightforward. We have a fairly clear idea of what it means to say that diseases are being prevented. By contrast neither the ends nor the means of 'well-being promotion' can be specified easily, or without controversy.

If we take well-being to include all of those things that make life 'go well', then 'the promotion of well-being' is a task seemingly without boundaries. This applies whether we think of well-being as something determined from an 'objective', external point of view or as something determined subjectively – by each individual making a judgement as to their level of well-being. In either case all kinds of things might be taken to contribute to a person's well-being: not only basic things like food, shelter and income; but also other fundamental building blocks like education, leisure, or personal and social relationships; and all kinds of relatively 'abstract' cultural and meaning-related goods such as art and religious belief. All these things, and all the environmental and social factors which underpin them, are relevant to the 'promotion of well-being'.

Given this compass for health promotion, it is not merely those people who contribute to disease prevention (plumbers etc.) who might be seen as health promoters but more or less anyone. The list of potential 'well-being' health promoters might include, for example, musicians, dating agencies, vicars, writers, film directors and so on – as well as those we more often think of as promoting health. And we should note that these people would not just qualify as potential health promoters because their activities might indirectly prevent disease (e.g. by improving mood and thereby boosting the immune system); they would be health promoters by dint of their direct effects. If we equate health with well-being, then a piano teacher who had the effect of making a pupil appreciate and enjoy music (and thereby contributed to the quality of their life) would, in that way, be directly promoting health. Some people may feel that this stretches the meaning of health to the point of absurdity: that there must be some middle ground between, on the one hand, equating health with the absence of disease; and on the other, with complete well-being. We will come back to this idea of a compromise shortly. First, we need to say a little more about the broad idea of well-being.

Even this brief discussion of these two senses of health is enough to indicate that as we go from the narrow to the broader sense of health something else happens. We move from a sense of health which is essentially defined in expert terms and typically in ways which derive from the clinical sciences; to a sense in which health is much more open-ended and contested. This is not to suggest that there cannot be disputes or disagreements about the definition or ascription of disease – it is important to see that these expert-led questions can themselves be subject to debate and controversy. It is rather to emphasise the sheer scope of potential disagreement and diversity when we move to talk about well-being. In other words, while we do not want to imply that those who rely on a narrow conception of health can thereby treat it as a value-free concept; a construction of health which broadly equates it with well-being makes health unequivocally and wholly a value-laden issue (Downie, Tannahill & Tannahill 1996). There is so much potential for disagreement about the relative importance of various components of well-being, and to an important degree there is potential for disagreement about whether or not something is a component of well-being in the first place. Not everyone would think that having a lot of money, or having a strong religious faith contributed to well-being, but for some people one or other of these things might appear central to achieving well-being. Someone who wanted to promote well-being would have to be very careful not to make assumptions about what exactly to promote.

Some writers have attempted to find a middle way between the very narrow and very broad conceptions of health we have just described. They have tried to capture the idea that health is a basic condition for well-being but is not equivalent to well-being itself. For example, Seedhouse (2001) has summarised health as 'the foundations for achievement'; while Nordenfelt (1987) has talked of it as 'the ability to achieve vital goals', adding that this conception is not a new one but can be found in the writing of authors both ancient and modern. The accounts from the two writers we have just mentioned form part of a philo-sophical debate about the nature of health. Similar 'middle way' conceptions of health can, though, be found in less theoretical contexts such as the WHO's more recent characterisation of health as 'a resource for living' (World Health Orga-nisation 1986). While these various 'middle way' accounts are doubtless impor-tantly different from each other in some respects; what they have in common is that they see health as more than the absence of disease and less than open-ended well-being. Health is the capacity to achieve well-being. In other words, we attain a state of health to the extent that we have the resources to be able to live a fulfilling life. Whether we then go on to live a fulfilling life (or exactly how we define a fulfilling life) is not the point. According to these 'middle way' con-ceptions, health care is about meeting people's basic needs and thereby providing the conditions for their personal autonomy. This includes controlling the effects of diseases; but it also includes the requirement to provide or facilitate other necessary resources such as information, or supportive relationships. A health promoter may be better placed to make some broad assumptions about what kinds of basic resources people might need without necessarily knowing much about their individual conceptions of well-being.

Our primary interest here is not to compare and evaluate rival conceptions of health. We are simply illustrating some of the elasticity of health promotion. This 'middle way' picture would entail that health promotion meant something like promotion of 'the conditions for autonomy' (which we understand here to mean the capacity to live one's life in the way one wants). Our point is not whether this is a plausible, or defensible, picture of health promotion. (Although we should note in passing that many people will also find this too broad a picture because it effectively breaks what they see as the necessary link between disease and health.) We are not interested in trying to solve some abstract puzzle about the meaning of expressions. However, we are interested in highlighting the ambiguities that exist here and in stressing the need for health promoters to be reflective about the way in which they (and the people around them) use the language of health promotion. It is essential for health promoters to recognise the debates sur-rounding the notion of health and the implications this has for the project of promoting health.

We have pointed towards three broad pictures of health: the absence of disease; well-being; and the 'middle way' of health as a condition for well-being. Of course, individuals (and communities) will also have their own understandings of health and illness which will cut across these broad pictures. Given this, no health promoter can simply characterise their objective as promoting 'health'. Unless they have a more precise account of what this actually means as an objective, no-one will know what they are trying to do! We will return to this theme later on in the book.

For the time being though, it is possible to say that in practice, those who work in the occupational field of health promotion have a wide range of objectives. A health promoter engaged in a particular intervention is likely to have a mix of objectives in undertaking that intervention. This is no different from most aspects of health care and indeed 'health promotion'-type objectives may often overlap with other sorts of health care objectives. For example, a nurse may work with a patient to get him to take his medicine, whilst at the same time helping him to feel physically comfortable, and also providing him with information and moral support with regard to preventing future disease episodes (or with regard to aspects of positive well-being). Quite often a specific disease-management focus is accompanied by a focus on other, broader, considerations, often called 'health promotion'. Typically, though, these broader considerations are anchored in some concern with disease management. In the real world of health promotion as an occupation (or part of an occupation), it might perhaps be odd to see anything included which was not – in some respect – anchored in disease management.

Health promotion – values and ethics

In practice, the issue about the goals of health promotion is less 'What conception of health is being applied?' and more 'What mix of ends is being pursued and what is the relative priority attached to these different ends?'. If different sorts of ends are being pursued, there is more than a fair chance of conflict between them and in these cases we have to ask a further question; 'How are these different sorts of ends to be reconciled?'. Responses to this question cannot remain only at the practical level – do more of A in some circumstances and less of B, say, or concentrate on Y with a particular target group and on Z with another. This is because the conflict is not just practical or technical; it is also one of values. We should be concerned to ask what ought to be our ends in undertaking health promotion as well as how those ends are being or might be achieved.

This distinction between what actually happens or might happen in practice and what ought to happen is straightforward and familiar, but it is vital. We all make this distinction on a day-to-day basis when we criticise the conventions, routines and assumptions of the settings in which we live and work. A nurse being inducted into a new ward would be failing in her duty if she did not question what she saw as bad or ethically unacceptable practice merely because it happened to be normal practice. In the same way the 'evaluation' of health promotion should never be simply a judgement about whether an intervention *works on its own terms.* A programme designed forcibly to sterilise all homeless people so that they will not bring homeless and therefore, at-risk, babies in the world might be 100% successful on its own terms – but that would not make it a real success. The legitimacy, both of conceptions of 'effectiveness' and of methods used, needs to be brought under the scope of evaluation. Although this is obviously an extreme example, we should be deeply sceptical about any supposed evaluation which neglects these issues. In fact, we suggest, we should withhold the label of evaluation from them.

We will say more about the distinctiveness of value and ethical issues in health promotion in the next chapter and throughout the book. But it is important to emphasise at this point that these issues are not new. Health promotion's discussion about values is long-standing. It forms part of the 'models debate' (Beattie 1991, Downie, Tannahill & Tannahill 1996, Ewles & Simnett 1995, Tones 1983, 1990) which we have obliquely encountered in this chapter. People new to the field sometimes make the mistake of thinking this debate is merely about the technical effectiveness of different approaches. What is the best technique: is it to encourage people to comply with medical advice; or to simply give them information; or to build their skills and confidence; or to enable community action; or to change policies, structures and environments etc.? But, of course, these debates are not essentially about technique. They are about what should be seen as valuable and acceptable in health promotion. Which ends are most important? Where are the best places to intervene? When, and to what extent, is it justifiable to place responsibility in the hands of individuals, or local communities, or governments? Is it fair to put pressure on individuals in order to improve their health or the health of the population? These are the broad questions at the heart of this debate about models – and at the heart of health promotion ethics.

For the rest of the book, we will largely avoid debates about the meaning and scope of health promotion. We will take health promotion to refer to the work of those people who think of themselves as working as health promoters. As we have noted this does not necessarily pick out a coherent body of work, or of approaches to work, because the term is a slippery one which people use in different ways. This elasticity is arguably one of the reasons the term has been so successful. It holds together the rather different interests and concerns of people with quite separate perspectives. It is a suitable banner under which these different groups can make common cause and appeal both to policy makers and to the whole population – who, after all, could be against the promotion of health? The banner is effective, in part, because it masks the disagreements of those who gather under it. But it wouldn't work at all if it was completely meaningless. Health promotion, we have seen, is a label which is used to pick out work for health which transcends curative health care. It encompasses work aimed at the prevention of disease and work aimed at the promotion of 'positive health'. In general this work is well intentioned, embodies widely-held values and has important goals, but none of this is enough. Health promotion demands ethical scrutiny and justification.

Chapter 2
The Challenge to Professional Ethics

Wider and deeper health work

We have seen that health promotion represents a broad approach to health care. On the one hand, it shares with the public health tradition what might be called a 'wide' focus – that is to say, an interest in the determinants and consequences of diseases. Whereas therapeutic health care concentrates mainly on a relatively short causal chain – that between treatment and cure – public health has an interest in a much longer one which includes the natural history and social effects of diseases. On the other hand, health promotion, like a number of other trends in health care, has what might be called a focus on 'depth': that is to say, a concern not only with the causes and consequences of disease; but also with the experiences, perceptions, choices and quality of life of individuals and groups. To some extent, these concerns with width and depth conflict with each other. The latter concern tends to be presented as a rejection of the medical model; whereas the former is essentially an extension of it. The former might be called the 'hard' face of health promotion, to be distinguished from the latter 'soft' face. At various places in this book, we will come back to the tensions between these two faces. The main purpose of this chapter, however, is to introduce the implications of this broad – both wide and deep – approach for the professional ethics of those engaged in health promotion work.

Health promotion involves new and extended roles, new spheres of concern and new sorts of work. All of these have important implications for health professionals and health care ethics. They all raise fundamental questions about both the 'ends' and the 'means' of health care. We will briefly sketch these changes in practical terms before going on to draw out their importance for values and ethics.

First, health promotion is changing the job descriptions, and so the self-understanding of many health professionals. Dentists, doctors, nurses, pharmacists and many others are being encouraged to think of themselves as health promoters – to have regard to ways of supporting the longer-term health and well-being of their clients. (See, for example, Scriven & Orme (2001) for an elucidation of a number of professional roles in relation to the promotion of health.) This entails taking an interest in the ongoing life circumstances of their clients and potential clients: the settings in which they live and work; their habits, beliefs about health, and personal preferences. (Although we recognise some difficulties with it, we will generally use the term 'clients' when referring to those who are served by health promoters and health promotion specialists. If we are talking about nurses and doctors serving people in specific health care settings, we will sometimes use the term 'patient', as this seems most natural in such a context.) Second, there are now some roles devoted wholly to health promotion – roles which we are labelling as health promotion specialist. These individuals are not 'extending' their roles into new 'wider' and 'deeper' spheres with particular clients. Rather, they are interested primarily in developing and underpinning the infrastructure of health – that is to say, in helping build healthier communities and settings and so supporting individual efforts to live healthier lives. Third, both health promoters and health promotion specialists are, as a result, extending health work's spheres of concern. When faced with clients, often they not only 'focus in' on habits, body systems, organs etc., they also 'focus out' onto people's whole life experience and the physical and cultural contexts which shape lives. Finally, the means employed by health promoters are different in kind to those employed in 'curative care'. You cannot work on community development or environmental change with the tools or knowledge derived, for example, from surgery or pharmacology. Different kinds of knowledge and tools are required.

We hope it is clear – even on the basis of this very short summary – that these changes add up to a very different agenda for some health professionals. They change the ways in which these people think about their roles, what they do in practice and the experiences and expectations of their clients. They create new sets of professional roles and relationships. As we will illustrate, these re-orientations cause similar re-orientations in professional ethics. It is not only that a whole lot of specific ethical issues and dilemmas are created by the health promotion movement; but also that this movement raises basic questions about the relationships between health professionals, their clients and society as a whole. Furthermore, these changes are taking place at a time when, as mentioned in the previous chapter, the whole basis and rationale of professional roles and professionalism is already under strain. The 'new' practices demanded by health promotion are taking place in changed professional contexts.

In order to illustrate the challenge which health promotion poses to professional ethics, we will rely on a rather exaggerated distinction between health promotion and other facets of health care. In the following section we will contrast health promotion ethics and health care professional ethics across a number of dimensions. In each case we are rather stretching the differences and, in effect, using 'ideal types' which do not correspond exactly with the much more complex and messy reality. Nonetheless, we want to maintain that the broad outline of the distinctions we are making do reflect important differences in emphasis with key repercussions for professional ethics.

The challenges of health promotion for health professionals

For the purposes of presentation we will set out the implications of the distinctive nature of health promotion – distinctive, that is, from other facets of health care – under a number of headings:

- *proactive versus reactive health work*
- *the professional-client relationship*
- *the ends of health work*
- *the knowledge base for intervention.*

Of course, the factors discussed under these headings overlap and interact with one another. They are all connected because they are all products of the broadening of perspective which is characteristic of health promotion. After we have discussed them separately, we will also begin to explore their combined effects.

Proactive versus reactive health work

Suppose I injure my knee and go to see the GP or nurse practitioner at my local health centre. I enter the room, say 'hello' and 'I've hurt my knee, can you help?' As we all know – the familiarity of this process is important and something we will come back to – there will then follow a process of diagnosis leading to treatment, or at least onward referral for treatment. In essence the primary health care team, and anyone else they refer me to, will be responding to my concerns. I want my knee 'mended' and they will try to mend it – or facilitate this through referral. By presenting myself at the health centre I am doing a number of things: I am asking for help; I am defining the area where I need help; and I am giving whoever I see 'permission' to offer relevant help or advice. It would be reasonable to suppose, therefore, that the professional to whom I have chosen to present myself has a 'licence' to intervene in my life in certain qualified respects.

This can be demonstrated by considering some alternatives to the familiar process we have just described. First, suppose that on the way to the health centre a complete stranger comes up to me at the bus stop and says, 'I can see there's something wrong with your knee, take your trousers off and I'll have a look at it and see what I can do'. I might be pleased at such a display of public spirit but I would much more likely be confused, embarrassed and anxious. Second, suppose that when I present myself in the health centre and point out my knee the doctor or nurse says, 'Never mind about your knee – I have heard that you keep forgetting to help your children with their homework, and that you have a habit of blocking your neighbour's car in. You should make more of an effort to care about other people.' It may be that I would feel suitably chastised and leave feeling inclined to buck up my attitude and behaviour; but it is much more likely I would think this a gross invasion of my privacy and something which fell far outside the proper scope of the professional I went to see.

These two examples illustrate the importance of what we have called 'licence'; and the fact that this licence is circumscribed. As a society, and as individuals, we have reasonably defined expectations of the nature and scope of traditional health professional roles. We know roughly what to expect in general if we see a doctor or a nurse. Further, we have different and more specific expectations of such professionals depending on the setting in which they are working (for example, we give a different kind of licence to hospital staff than to primary health care staff). Most importantly, we suppose that in the main, health professional intervention is initiated by some kind of action and 'permission-giving' on our part. In the main, health care is reactive. It is a response on the part of health professionals to something that *we* start. This is not always the case of course. If we are injured and rendered unconscious by a road traffic accident we would not expect to have to initiate an intervention, and we would not expect the health professionals to wait for our permission. But the general point holds. (This 'exception' is not, in any case, very different from the example above: there is clearly something wrong that needs 'mending'; and – as this wording shows in itself – there is a clear set of societal expectations about what should happen. It might even be possible to say that health professionals have a standing, generalised 'permission' to intervene in these extreme circumstances.)

It should by now be starting to become clear why health promotion presents a challenge to professional ethics by virtue of the kind of work it aims to undertake. Both the 'widening' and the 'deepening' aspects of health promotion work create problems for our conventional expectations.

In terms of the 'widening' aspect. The attempt to intervene earlier in the causal chain of disease processes means that health promotion often entails interventions into the lives of well people, people who are going about their daily business with no thought that they may need 'help' from health professionals. In this way health promoters have to be proactive. They have to plan and organise interventions many of which are not prompted, or expected, by the people they are designed to benefit. From where do health promoters get their licence? What justifies their practice of interfering in people's lives in this fashion? How are they any different from the do-gooder who comes up to us at a bus stop?

The attempt to consider 'deeper' aspects of health or quality of life means that health promoters must take an interest in many things which go beyond 'disease management'. They might look at my knee and ask whether I am getting enough exercise, or exercising in the right way, or over-exercising; and what factors in my life are supporting me in, or hindering me from, living a well-balanced life. Am I depressed, am I eating properly, are my domestic circumstances happy, have I tried meditation etc.? At what point do they stray outside the licence I have granted them? Is it acceptable if I go with my injured knee and they spend most of the consultation trying to persuade me not to smoke? How is that different from them advising me to make more of an effort with my children's homework? Once they have moved away from the problem presented by the patient there appears to be no obvious dividing line between, say, persuasion on smoking and inquisition on my homework-helping practices.

The professional-client relationship

The nature of the work in which health promotion often tries to engage makes it clear that we need to re-think the nature of the relationship between the professional promoting health and their client. In a sense, this is a theme underlying the whole of the book. In this section we will confine ourselves to opening up just one major element of such re-thinking; namely, the difficulty of applying the notion of the professional-client relationship in the field of health promotion.

Because health promotion is largely concerned with creating the conditions for health for populations of people, it works on a very ambitious canvas. The whole of our physical and cultural environment is potentially subject to health promotion intervention. The sphere of potential action is immense and it is clearly far beyond the scope of individual practitioners working alone. In other words, effective health promotion depends not only on co-operation and teamwork; but also on wide-ranging, inter-sectoral, collaboration (Katz, Peberdy & Douglas 2001, Naidoo & Wills 1998). This is not to say that an individual health professional cannot 'do' health promotion. Rather it is to say that their success will typically also depend on the activities of others and not just on what they are able to undertake on their own. For example, the practice nurse at my local health centre might encourage me to adjust my lifestyle; but if the area I live in is very polluted and if there is nowhere I can go for affordable fruit and vegetables, the possibility of my changing is limited. Changing these environmental factors however, depends on concerted social action, work outside the reach of an individual practitioner.

There are, so to speak, 'three components' in the idea of the professional-client relationship: firstly, the professional; secondly, the client; and thirdly, the existence of a relationship between the two of these. But each of these components is not easily applied to health promotion. Who are the professionals? Who are the clients? What, if anything is the nature of the relationship between them? Whereas in the ideal type of conventional health care the professional-client relationship is essentially a real one-to-one, person-to-person, face-to-face relationship; none of these things need apply in health promotion. (Although, of course, they may sometimes.) Often, however, health promotion is implemented by large, sometimes diffuse, teams of people and is aimed at groups or populations. This is more of a teams-populations relationship than a person-to-person one. It is only a relationship, too, in the abstract sense that some people are implicated in other people's lives. There need be no mutual awareness between the parties of what is taking place. Take as an example a national campaign on healthy eating which involves media advertising, posters, and local action in hospitals and schools. Many of those behind the campaign will be invisible to the intended beneficiaries and *vice-versa*. It will be very difficult for the health promoters to trace out the effects of their actions on the intended beneficiaries; and similarly it will be very difficult for intended beneficiaries to trace back the lines of responsibility for the effects of the campaign. This is strikingly different from, say, hospital in-patient treatment where all the main 'players' are known to one another.

The example of the healthy eating campaign also serves to raise another question. Are all of the people involved in a campaign such as this properly described as 'professionals' in any case? Some of them may belong to recognised professional groups (for example, medicine and dentistry) and others may not; but even in the former case this does not seem to answer the question. Suppose your lawyer tells you that she is doing health promotion work in the evenings. Let us agree that by virtue of being a member of the legal profession, she is a professional. Does that mean we would see her as a professional with regard to her health promotion activity? Probably not. But are the doctors and dentists (and other health professionals) involved in the healthy eating campaign any different in this respect? If they extend their role in this way so that it encompasses health promotion, does this automatically make them health promotion professionals?

The ends of health work

Everything we have said up until now indicates that health promotion is connected to a revision of the goals – or the ends – of health-related work. This applies in relation to both its 'deepening' and its 'widening' facets. 'Deepening' orients work towards broader conceptions of health – for example, conceptions which link health with 'autonomy' or 'well-being'. 'Widening' prompts a move towards activity aimed at effecting the conditions for health, rather than responding to existing disease states. These two sets of factors, separately and combined, demand that health promoters take on board different ways of defining 'success'; and therefore different approaches to planning, implementing and evaluating their work. In this section, however, we want to concentrate not on these things – although they are fundamental – but on another equally central way in which health promoters have to question, and re-think, the ends of health work.

Given the issues discussed in the section above (the tendency for health promotion work to be proactive and aimed at populations), health promoters are faced with a key question: *Whose* health should be promoted? If there is a whole world of people whose health we might promote, where should we start? There will, of course, be some people who 'ask' us (one way or another) to promote their health. But this class of people is likely to be relatively small. There will be a much larger class of people who do not 'ask' for health promotion, but nevertheless we

– or policy-makers – believe that their health could be improved in some respects. To some extent this is not different from the sort of priority-setting dilemmas facing other health workers. A General Practitioner (GP) has to decide how to divide their time between the person they are currently seeing, patients queuing outside in the waiting room and patients needing attention at home. Should they spend so long talking to a man who is suffering from panic attacks when there is someone else who is in need of pain relief? But at least the GP's dilemmas are confined to the practice's list of patients. (And they are further focused by the fact that in the majority of cases, help has been requested.) The issue of priority-setting for a 'health promotion service' seems to be much more open-ended. How should it define and measure the need for health promotion? How should it determine which needs, and whose needs, are more pressing? How should it allocate its efforts, and other resources, to meet these needs fairly? These are clearly very difficult questions.

One way of capturing both the complexity and practical importance of this issue is to ask: what would count as equal access to health promotion; and how would we know if we had attained it? There are at least two plausible candidates for equal access models. However, the two models are very different indeed and tell different stories about the ends of health work. According to the first model, we might develop an indicator of equal access along these lines: a health promotion service provides equal access if efforts are made to try and ensure that potential beneficiaries of the service stand an equally good chance of benefiting from it in practice. Because of its concentration on ensuring processes are tailored to ensuring equality of access opportunity, we might call this a process model of equal access. Of course, such an indicator is certainly an important dimension of equity. It would entail, for example, that those organising a vaccination campaign would have to take care to have multiple translations of all their literature available; and they would need to conduct outreach work to at least make sure the information and resources that they had were available to those who didn't actively seek them. In short, a concern with equal access would entail a certain degree of 'targeting' of resources and effort. (In passing we should note that if such a service was really going to provide all relevant persons with an 'equal chance of benefiting' it would have to strongly skew its use of resources to the hard-to-reach groups with the likely result that the service would be less effective overall – simply because it was concentrating its work on a relatively small number of people.)

The second model potentially implies much more radical targeting practices. The argument for such a model might go along these lines: health promotion ought to aim at producing, insofar as this is possible, equal access to health itself and not just equal coverage of health promotion activities. Health promotion ought to be targeted so as to try to rectify existing experiences of unequal health. In its concern with the outcome of equal health (ignoring the difficulty in what this might actually mean), we can call this an outcome model of equal access. If in fact we put the emphasis on trying to reduce inequalities in health as this model suggests (and this, of course, is a goal close to the heart of many health pro-moters), then we would not primarily be concerned about achieving 'equal coverage' of health promotion work. We would regard it as much more impor-tant to 'raise the health stakes' for certain specific groups of people. The question of 'equal coverage' versus 'equal health' is only one dilemma – albeit an impor-tant one – related to 'the ends' of health promotion work. An array of others will be discussed later.

The knowledge base for intervention

In recent times, the knowledge base of health care has been put firmly on the policy agenda (Department of Health 1998). The evidence-based health care movement has put pressure on health professionals to question 'custom and practice' as a means of legitimising their interventions. Instead, they are being asked; How do you know this works? On close inspection it turns out, of course, that the knowledge base of many health care interventions is far from secure. In numerous instances there are uncertainties and disagreements about what works and about whether interventions are effective. The question, 'How do you know this works?', and the frequent difficulty in answering it convincingly, applies equally to health promotion (Perkins, Simnett & Wright 1999). However, it can be argued that health promoters face particular difficulties when it comes to providing a knowledge base for their activities. Moreover, these difficulties do not stem merely from the relatively 'young' nature of the field, and the con-sequent relative underdevelopment of its knowledge base, but more importantly from its essential character.

As we have seen, both the 'aims' and the methods of health promotion are more diffuse than those of curative health care. Although there is a lot of scope for disagreement about which (if any) treatment might be most effective for a particular disease; this scope magnifies considerably when we ask about effective health promotion. Partly this reflects the uncertainties that exist about what counts as health, or about the distribution of health promotion effort, which we have considered previously. Clearly, we cannot even begin to consider effec-tiveness of activity if our views on the ends of health promotion are unclear. However, even if we specify a determinate list of health promotion objectives, the problem remains. The underlying difficulty is that the underpinnings of health promotion are not supplied only by the biological and clinical sciences; but also by social sciences (Bunton & Macdonald 1992). Of course, the same can be said to some extent of all health professional work, particularly if we accept that the trends towards 'widening' and 'deepening' apply across all such work (Naidoo & Wills 2001). But the balance is crucially different in health promotion. And, for a number of reasons, the knowledge base of the social sciences is inherently contestable.

For example, a health promoter may use educational methods, legislation, or other public policy tools to achieve their goals. It is important to note that these sorts of methods are not merely accompaniments to the main processes of intervention but are in themselves the practices used to create change. Whereas doctors prescribing drugs will have to be sensitive to psychosocial processes (they cannot afford to ignore issues of accessibility or adherence for instance); psycho-social processes are frequently the principal route for the 'administration' of health promotion. More than this, health promotion typically aims at long-term change through the use of processes which are themselves both long-term and broad-ranging. The evidence base of health promotion depends therefore, on our knowledge of the effectiveness of such processes. So it is perhaps worth rehearsing briefly why this sort of knowledge is inherently uncertain and unreliable.

Social life forms an ever-changing open system in which many different kinds of things interact. It is not only that there are many variables; but also that the constantly changing interactions between them are very difficult to map. For example, what are the influences on the sexual behaviour of teenagers? How far should we consider, for instance, the effect of evolving gender roles, secularisation processes, changes in family structures and parental roles, the media and the effects of the market – just for example – on representations of sex and consequently on the sexual practices of young people? If we wish to intervene effectively, we will need at least to consider some of these things, the connections between them and the effect that our intervention will have when added to this compound of social processes. This task is clearly a demanding one. Moreover, the problem is contributed to by the fact that social life is constantly evolving. Just because a particular type of intervention appeared to be effective on one occasion, it does not follow that it will have the same effects again. Cultural, social and environmental changes mean that the sorts of generalisations which are possible in biological sciences do not apply. There is, then, a real difficulty in achieving what is called 'predictive validity' in the social sciences; that is to say, of being able to make confident claims about the effects of our interventions.

So health promoters – especially where they have ambitious aims for improving public health – face a huge challenge. Do they have the necessary knowledge to achieve their objectives? Why should society even contemplate accepting the existence of health promotion activities if health promoters are often unclear about whether what they are doing is likely to have good or bad effects, or even any effect at all?

A different sort of health work

The relative emphasis on proactive intervention, the focus on populations, and the open-ended nature of the goals and methods of health promotion all combine to make it what we might reasonably call a different sort of health work. In this section we will reflect further on the distinctiveness of health promotion interventions. In doing this, we also want to add an explicit note about something which has been largely implicit until now – that is to say, the overlap between health promotion and politics.

Accepting that health promoters have more or less ambitious objectives: and that some work may be relatively modest both in scope and aim; in overall terms, it would be quite reasonable to claim that health promotion is about social action for social benefit. It cannot, then, be insulated from the public world or debates about the public interest. It overlaps conspicuously with both practical politics and political philosophy. (Other aspects of health care are also implicated with politics, of course. However, they can frequently give the impression of being insulated from it – although we would want to emphasise that this is only an impression.) In other words health promoters have, to some extent, to engage in political activity to achieve their ends; and health promotion approaches inevitably have built into them assumptions about political philosophy. These include, for example, assumptions about the nature of a just society, or about the legitimacy of state (or professional) intervention into people's lives and life circumstances. (See Kelly (1996) for an interesting example of critique on some dominant health promotion assumptions. Of course Kelly also demonstrates his own political stance.)

It is understandable that some health professionals say they are interested in helping people – but that they are not interested in politics. We may think this short-sighted or muddle-headed, but we can understand what they mean. However it makes absolutely no sense for someone to say they are interested in health promotion, but not in politics. If politics is about the collective ways in which we decide upon, and organise, the conditions of our society then you might even say that health promotion is a form of politics. It is inextricably linked to it in a variety of ways; and political activity is one of the tools of health promotion (Rodmell & Watt 1986).

This overlap with politics is a further example of the distinctiveness of health promotion. It stems from the fact that health promotion interventions are often broader in scope and work through a range of social axes. Face-to-face interventions are usually set in the context of programmes which work through – or emerge from – public policies and institutions. Every kind of 'axis of influence' is relevant. Health promotion can use physical mechanisms (for example, fluoridation and vaccination); 'threats' and incentives (such as legislation and economic measures); and 'cultural engineering' (for example, peer pressure and social marketing); as well as more person-centred approaches like counselling and education (Downie, Tannahill & Tannahill 1996). These different forms of influence give rise to distinctive ethical issues; for example, when, if ever, is it justifiable to coerce someone to change their behaviour in order to improve their own health, or someone else's health? Similarly, questions about the proper use of the law, or public policy, or environmental intervention 'in the cause of health' raise complex ethical problems which transcend the typical agenda of medical or nursing ethics. The central focus of this book is the ethical dilemmas faced by individual health promoters, so we will not be considering these public policy questions in any depth. They will, however, form a necessary part of the background to our discussions. Sometimes, indeed, they may appear to occupy the foreground. This is because the impact of policy on the work of individual health promoters is on occasions very substantial indeed.

Implications for professional ethics

One implication of the above discussion is that we should perhaps place the expression 'professional ethics' in inverted commas when it is applied to health promotion. There is neither a clear-cut profession of health promoters; nor a model of the professional-client relationship which is of obvious relevance. We could say that this is a book about 'practitioner ethics' in the occupational field of health promotion. That, though, seems to be too much of a mouthful, so we will stick with the term 'professional ethics' despite our qualifications and concerns about the applicability of the term in the context of health promotion. However we must stress that the expression is only being used loosely. In particular, we would not wish to let the mere use of the expression 'professional' confer any sense of legitimacy or ethical acceptability on health promotion activities. Whether or not these activities are ethically justifiable or acceptable cannot turn on their simple labelling as professional activities. This may seem obvious, but the fact that the label 'professional' does itself seem to carry some ethical weight is important – and something which we want to explore a little further as a means of pulling the threads of this chapter together.

Health care professionals such as doctors and nurses are called professionals not only because they belong to certain occupational groups; but also because they are expected to display certain sorts of standards. (The next two paragraphs are based upon the analysis of Daryl Koehn in The Ground of Professional Ethics (Koehn 1994). We have discussed the relevance of this work for health promotion elsewhere (Cribb & Duncan 1999); here we will merely summarise that discussion.) A typical summary account of the nature of professional groups is to say that they emerge from a contract or bargain between an occupational group and the wider society it aims to serve. The occupational group concerned gets some degree of control over the field in which they work and, in return, they guarantee certain technical and ethical standards. No-one can just call themselves a doctor or a nurse – they have to earn these roles by following certain educational and professional paths. These roles are defined and safeguarded by professional bodies underpinned by the authority of the state. Other members of society are thereby, at least to some degree, curtailed from practising in these fields. However – as a consequence of this curtailment – they have *prima facie* grounds to place their trust in the doctors and nurses with whom they come into contact.

The professional-client relationship is built upon this wider societal bargain. This bargain is what lies behind the definite, but circumscribed, licence we give to the professionals with whom we deal. If I go to see a doctor, for example, I go with a set of expectations about what the doctor is there for; how they will behave, and what is expected of me. (Recall the example, earlier in the chapter, of the injured knee.) In particular, I go with the reasonable expectation that they will be committed to applying their expertise to the resolution of my medical problems. This is a perfectly reasonable expectation as this professional commitment will normally have been 'lived out' in the doctor's words and deeds for a considerable time; it is implicit in their 'professing' to be a doctor. (This also helps explain our justified anger, and horror, on those occasions when this expectation turns out to be misplaced.)

The background societal bargain is reinforced by the particular agreements that occur when I give my explicit or implicit 'permission' for the doctor to offer advice and treatment; and when actually faced with a suggested course of action I have another chance to agree – to give my informed consent – to a particular course of action. These levels of expectation and agreement serve to underpin, and are an expression of, the professional-client relationship. They also help to shed light on the 'ethical weight' of the idea of the professional. The fact that we associate professionals with good practice and high ethical standards is understandable. However, we cannot rely on these associations to legitimate health promotion work: partly because, as we have discussed, health promotion cannot be conceived of as a profession; and partly because the associations by themselves are not enough to confer ethical authority on activity. (This latter reason means, of course, that it can never be enough for even an established profession, for example, medicine, to claim it is ethical simply because it is a profession. We would need to look much more carefully at the kinds of licence sought and given both in general and in particular cases.)

So, if health promoters cannot derive their 'ethical licence' from the social conventions and agreements that underpin most health care professionalism what should they do? What are the lessons of this chapter for the 'professional ethics' of health promotion?

First, it is essential that health promoters are conscious of the issues we have outlined here. In particular they have to be aware of the absence of a clear social licence for their work. This awareness points in two directions. On the one hand, it will encourage a healthy scepticism about the legitimacy of their own activities; and on the other hand, it will point to the need to negotiate agreement and broad 'consent', at least to the extent that this is possible. Both of these things indicate the importance of conducting health promotion 'in the public domain' – that is to say, of making it as open to public inspection and participation as possible and of treating the views of individuals and communities with respect.

Second, the absence of traditional professional structures and practices in most areas of health promotion, and the fact that health promotion is spread across different contexts and institutions, places a lot of responsibility on each individual to critically examine the work in which they are implicated. Because no-one in particular is easily identifiable as being responsible for large scale programmes, health promoters have a duty to ensure that each and every one of them takes ethical responsibility rather than no-one at all. (Of course, this should be true of all health professionals but in many roles and institutional settings there are tight forms of supervision and safety nets which arguably makes this level of self-scrutiny less crucial.) Above all, health promoters cannot afford to accept that because some authoritative agency or person says that something is a worthwhile project, it must therefore be worthwhile and ethically acceptable. It can only be judged worthwhile if it is looked at and the values that are built into its goals and strategies are subjected to questioning.

Third, health promoters need to look 'widely and deeply' for potential ethical problems in all aspects of their own work and its effects. In particular they must be sensitive to the fact that intervening in personal and social processes raises at least as many ethical issues as intervening in biological processes. For example, simply because something is called 'education', it does not automatically follow that it is ethically neutral or ethically praiseworthy. We have to look at exactly what happens in practice. Is a health promoter who 'informs' someone about a screening programme actually putting pressure on them (directly or indirectly) to comply with the aims and procedures of the programme? Is the health promoter who is 'encouraging' new mothers to consider the advantages of breast feeding actually stigmatising those who cannot or would prefer not to? (Of course, it may be that on occasions these sorts of pressures can be ethically justified – this possibility also needs consideration.)

Finally, and most importantly, health promoters need to incorporate the language of values and ethics into their day to day practice. Many do so already but it is essential that it becomes as commonplace as talking about 'effectiveness' or 'evaluation'. Indeed evaluation cannot take place, nor can effectiveness be properly assessed, unless ethics is considered. For all of the reasons set out above, ethics must become a staple in the conversations of health promoters. The issues in health promotion ethics are too complex for them to be considered by individuals in isolation. They require continuous dialogue and debate if health promoters are going to be sufficiently aware of, and responsive to, all of their implications; and are able to build better checks and balances into the occupational field of health promotion.

In Section Two and Section Three of the book we hope to help contribute towards these developments. In Section Two we will concentrate on exploring some of the ethical issues facing health promoters. It is not possible to deal with the whole range of issues so we have chosen some indicative examples. The section is organised so that each of its four chapters has both a theoretical and a practical theme. These themes provide the overarching framework of the discussion but within this framework we will also explore a number of related issues and further develop the arguments of the book as a whole. The emphasis of Section Two is on elaborating the value and ethical issues rather than upon trying to resolve them. As we have just indicated, one of our working assumptions is that progress can be made simply by putting these issues firmly on the agenda of health promoters, eliciting their dimensions and implications, and encouraging dialogue and reflection about them. Section Three, however, turns to the question of how practitioners might at least make some progress with 'resolving' the ethical issues of health promotion, or at least with 'managing' them skilfully and responsibly. In Section Three we will consider the different kinds of resources health promoters can turn to for help.

There are no easy answers to the questions of health promotion ethics. Indeed, it may sometimes seem that there are no answers at all. One of the characteristics of all ethical questions is that there is no agreed formula to which we can turn for a definitive answer. This can have the effect of inducing a sense that the questions are simply 'impossible' and therefore no point can be found in discussing them. We believe the opposite. The questions may sometimes seem impossibly complex and difficult but they are inescapable. The way in which health promoters work, and the programmes they implement, are based upon 'answers' to value and ethical questions. The only options are whether health promoters 'answer' these questions knowingly and thoughtfully or unknowingly and thoughtlessly.

Section Two
Values and Ethics in Health Promotion Practice

Introduction to Section Two

Up to now we have been treating health promotion as a specific kind of occupational practice, and have used this approach to avoid some of the more abstract and slippery questions about the nature of health promotion. We continue this pragmatic approach in this section of the book and ask – *What kinds of value judgements and ethical issues are attached to the work of health promoters?*

Inevitably, we cannot discuss this question in relation to every kind of activity in which a health promoter might be involved. Even as a specific occupational practice, health promotion involves a multitude of things. We have however, chosen some examples that represent a range of health promotion work. Part of the rationale for the choice of examples is that they can be used to illustrate a key values-related issue that appears again and again in health promotion. For example, in Chapter Three, we discuss health behavioural counselling and face-to-face education. This kind of work raises an important ethical tension for those promoting health: is it about empowering people; or is it about controlling them? But this tension does not only occur in this kind of work. It runs across a huge swathe of health promotion activity, from policy development to community participation. We have chosen the 'case study' to exemplify a wider ethical issue, and this rationale applies to all the other cases we examine. Also in the exploration of each of the central issues, we identify other ethical and values-related tensions, frequently overlapping within and across the chapters. It is hard to avoid the impression of a spider's web of difficulties being exposed.

But unless issues are identified and mapped we cannot even begin to deal with them. In Section Three, we consider this task of dealing with the ethical difficulties of health promotion. For now, we simply explore the issues in the hope of encouraging greater awareness about values and ethics. We will be asking about the values embodied in different approaches to health promotion, and seeking to clarify and map some of the central value judgements inherent in the occupational field. In so doing we will also begin to explore the defensibility of these different value sets so that we can work towards the 'ethical assessment' of health promotion practice.

Values in practice

In the previous section, we hope to have made clear a number of fundamental issues related to health promotion and professional practice. We began by arguing that health promotion can be understood as one response to changing perspectives on health care at the turn of the millennia. These changing perspectives include increased focus on client – or person – centred health care; greater emphasis on recognising and understanding the social and environmental determinants of health; and increased weight being placed on broader and more flexible notions of the nature of health and well-being. Against these has emerged what we are thinking of as a specific kind of occupational practice – health promotion.

We also discussed the idea that different people understand health promotion as having different aims. For example: to prevent disease; to promote well-being; to provide 'resources for living'. Because the aims of health promotion work are disputed and value-laden, their examination is a fundamental first stage in the process of value clarification and ethical assessment. If we are unclear about an activity's aim or purpose, how can we begin to make ethical judgements related to it? An example will help illustrate this. Imagine that an NHS hospital trust implements a no smoking policy on its premises. The aim of this may be to do with disease prevention (reducing the incidence of smoking will, in some way, lower levels of smoking-related ill health and disease). Or the aim may be to support those trust employees that are trying to break the habit. There may be a range of other, health-related aims for this piece of work. This might make it attractive to a number of different 'values camps' within health promotion. But it could equally be the case that in the examination of aim, we detect a strong preference on the part of the NHS trust for its aim to be prevention of disease. This might make some – the 'well-being' health promoters – less likely to view the activity sympathetically.

So far, we have only considered the health-related aims for this activity. In Chapter Two, we made it clear that there was a strong overlap between health promotion and politics. Health promotion aims – in important respects, the aims of political policy – can be intertwined with other policy aims. Indeed, the aims of health promotion can on occasion – possibly frequently – be subsumed into other, non-health, policy aims (Wikler 1978).

What do we mean by this? Sticking with the example of the NHS trust implementing a no smoking policy, it could be that the trust managers are alarmed at the prospect of an employee suing the organisation at some point in the future for damages related to ill-health due to passive smoking. Thus their primary aim in introducing the smoking policy is to avoid litigation and protect the finances of the trust. Of course, it may be very hard for an outsider to discover this is the managers' primary aim, they are far more likely to talk about health-related aims. It is clear, too, that this non-health related aim could co-exist with what will most likely be the explicit health aim or aims of the work. These two sets of aims represent very different sets of values.

Earlier we made it clear that from different conceptions of health promotion and its aims also emerge views on the appropriateness of separate *approaches* to the promotion of health. Examining the approach of health promoters as they undertake a particular activity is therefore another necessary element of values clarification and ethical assessment. But there will be multiple accounts available here also.

Another example will help to illustrate this. Bob Jones is a 38 year old man admitted to a hospital surgical ward for investigations related to gastric pain. These reveal acute gastritis, which is treated medically. On admission, history-taking reveals Mr Jones to be a heavy drinker – four pints of beer a night or the equivalent of 56 units of alcohol a week – well over the recommended 'safe limits' (Health Education Authority 1993). The staff nurse on duty at the time of Mr Jones' discharge takes the opportunity to speak to him about his drinking before he leaves the hospital's care. There are at least two kinds of approaches the staff nurse might take. The first would be something like this. The staff nurse is alarmed at Mr Jones' heavy drinking and believes the gastritis could be an 'early warning' for much more serious disease and possibly premature mortality. She warns him of this in very clear terms and strongly encourages him to reduce his alcohol intake, if not to try and give up altogether. The second approach might centre around a more open-ended discussion of Mr Jones' current drinking, asking him how he sees his drinking pattern, what might be the reasons for his heavy drinking, whether he has considered cutting down and what support he might need if he were to try and do so. Broadly speaking, the first approach operates according to the so-called 'medical model' – there is a problem here, recognised by 'the experts', that will lead to disease and should be prevented. Prevention, of course, may well be a motivator in the second approach, but here the direction taken could be seen as being much more 'client-centred'.

These approaches represent different sets of values. Included in the first are the values of 'expert' advice, of patient compliance with this and so on. In the second, amongst others, are the values of focusing on the patient, listening to what he is saying and allowing him to make his own judgements. Both of these approaches might result in behaviour change (and therefore the possibility of disease prevention). But, independently of this, it is possible to imagine there being disagreement about which approach is better from an ethical point of view – does one of them treat Mr Jones with more respect than the other? Does one of them show more concern to improve Mr Jones' welfare than the other?

It is, of course, possible to argue that certain work simply shouldn't be done at all. In Chapter Two, we argued that health promotion represented a challenge to traditional ways of thinking about the ethics of professional activity. In general, mainstream health care is reactive, circumscribed and licensed. In the case of Mr Jones, it might be argued that he has sought the help of health care professionals for his gastritis and any attempt – whether 'medical model' or 'client-centred' – to get him to think about his heavy drinking is stretching the licence he has given to those professionals. Of course, the professionals concerned could reply that there is a strong likelihood that Mr Jones' gastric symptoms have been caused by his heavy drinking. This may in fact be the case, but proving that there were causal connections between one and the other may be very hard – what other parts of the patient's medical history have been left relatively unexplored as a result of the preoccupation with his heavy drinking? There might be good reason for dealing with Mr Jones' heavy drinking as part of a plan for treating the gastritis, but equally there might not.

Another argument we advanced for the challenge offered by health promotion to professional ethics also has relevance here. We suggested (again in Chapter Two) that while some health promotion interventions are conducted 'face-to-face' between patients or clients and health professionals, many are not. In Mr Jones' case, such a face-to-face relationship clearly exists. There is the possibility of the staff nurse being able to pick up cues or explicit statements from the patient that he is unhappy with her approach; and for her to modify it or abandon it completely. But this can't be the case in interventions where there is no face-to-face relationship between those planning and delivering health promotion work, and those receiving it. The policy makers planning an approach to, say, improved dental health through fluoridation of an area's water supplies are in this sort of position. How far can real consent be obtained here – from a whole population – and if it cannot then perhaps this sort of health promotion work cannot be ethically legitimised at all?

One way of resisting this assertion is to point to the aim or aims of the work, and to the good consequences intended to follow from it. At least one of the aims of fluoridation is an improvement in the dental health of a population through reducing the incidence of caries (British Fluoridation Society 1996). This aim might satisfy quite a broad range of people with different perceptions of the nature of health promotion, as it relates to disease prevention directly and well-being indirectly. But does fluoridation actually prevent caries and so improve dental health? This is a question of *effectiveness* of health promotion work; and considering knowledge of effectiveness is another necessary element of values clarification and ethical assessment. Of course, just as the consideration of aims and approach is contested so is the consideration of effectiveness.

Even assuming the simple model of health promotion as disease prevention we run into problems straight away. First, there is the difficulty that in relation to much health promotion work, we simply do not know whether it is effective at preventing disease. Here, the problem is partly that of connecting a specific intervention with a particular health outcome. If the occurrence of caries is reduced and dental health improves in a given population, how do we know that these are the outcomes of fluoridation? There are a large number of other factors which might have contributed to the outcome or even been its principle cause –

for example, changes in population diet over time, uptake of preventive dental services and demographic shifts. Suggesting that a health promotion action caused a particular disease prevention is in many cases extremely problematic and the techniques employed by researchers to examine disease prevention in relation to mainstream medical interventions may simply not be suited to most health promotion (Webb 1999). This problem applies to the whole range of health promotion work and not just to policy intervention at population level. For example, even if we were able to find out that Mr Jones had, at some future point, cut down on his heavy drinking, how could we know that this was due to the staff nurse's particular intervention? As we have already remarked, there are substantial methodological problems in tracking long-term psychosocial processes.

The situation is complicated enormously if we think of health promotion as broader than disease prevention – for example, as encompassing the promotion of well-being or encouraging empowerment. These other ways of thinking about health promotion imply alternative versions of 'effectiveness'. The problem now is not simply one of measurement – of knowing how and whether we have been effective – but also of knowing exactly what 'effectiveness' is. What most contributes to 'well-being', say, for Mr Jones? Is it no further attacks of gastritis? Is it cutting down or giving up drinking? Is it carrying on drinking? Dispute, disagreement and doubt amongst health promoters therefore operate at the connected levels of professional 'ideology' and practice: of deciding what counts as evidence; and of deciding how what counts should actually be measured or otherwise assessed.

Ethical assessment

All of this contestability creates even more complexity and uncertainty and raises the question of whether the process of values clarification is a help or a hindrance to practice. As we have seen there are multiple 'accounts' in health promotion. We would argue that there is a need to find a way of examining these multiple accounts, differentiating between them and evaluating their respective claims. If we do not, there is a risk that we will become complacent or 'ethically blind'. We might end up believing, as some writers on health promotion have suggested, that any activity is acceptable so long as it works (Ewles & Simnett 1995). To us, this position is untenable. If we only see an activity on its own terms, and fail to judge whether we consider it corresponding with values that we consider to be ethically defensible, then as we have already said, there are ultimately no constraints on action. Think back to our example in Chapter One of the programme designed forcibly to sterilise all homeless people so that they will not bring homeless, at risk, babies into the world. Here, aim and approach could conspire to make such a programme 100% 'effective'. But would we be happy with this programme? Would it constitute 'good practice'? Rigorous ethical assessment of our work provides us with an essential way of reflecting on what both we, and others, do. In a contested field, it is a pre-requisite for defending our work.

So far we have talked about the need to reflect upon the aims, approach and knowledge of effectiveness of health promotion interventions. As we have stressed, the investigation of the facts and the mapping of the values needed for ethical assessment is often enormously complex and contested: but it is nevertheless possible to imagine a good deal of clarity about an intervention; and yet for dispute about what *ought* to be done to continue. There is, for example, reasonable evidence about the effect of prolonged and heavy drinking on susceptibility to disease. The approach of the staff nurse to Mr Jones may be one of concern and respect. The nurse's aim may be solely to improve the patient's welfare. Despite all this reassurance, however, we can still imagine someone prepared to assert that intervening is wrong. The kind of argument that might be put forward against intervention is so familiar we can almost hear it: Mr Jones' life is his own: he came into hospital for very specific treatment; we are no more than agents for a 'nanny state' if we start to interfere in how he lives. It is quite possible to make, and argue for, conflicting value judgements. (In this case, for example, the value of preventing disease on the one hand; *versus* the value of limiting professional involvement where this has not specifically been sought on the other.)

But from where do we derive the frameworks of values against which we make ethical judgements about examples of health promotion? This is a highly controversial question (and a question about which there are extensive debates which fall outside the scope of this book). Certain values are so deeply embedded in our cultural life that we tend to take them for granted, they are 'common sense' and we are also quite used to identifying tensions between them. We may not express these tensions as ethical dilemmas, or use ethically charged vocabulary to describe them, but we recognise them in practice (the tension between preventing harm and non-paternalism mentioned above is a case in point). But 'common sense' values and value frameworks are also subject to challenge and critique. In our own comparatively recent history, gender inequality was part of our taken for granted value framework. Those with an academic interest in ethics seek to articulate and defend value frameworks. In so doing they both draw upon and critique our common sense assumptions about values. (This process is discussed more fully in Section Three.) Although there is considerable disagreement amongst ethicists as to the best frameworks for ethical assessment, what they share in common is equally important. Namely the need:

(1)   to be explicit about the value framework against which ethical judgements are made; and
(2)   the need to be able to explain and defend the use of this value framework.

In our discussion thus far we have relied upon some widespread intuitions about ethics. We have, for example, mentioned the idea that clients may be entitled to non-interference from health professionals, and that there would be something wrong about a health promoter proceeding without the agreement of their clients. We have also suggested that some interventions (perhaps fluoridation) may be justifiable because they lead to such valuable consequences. These different intuitions – that ethics is about not breaching certain sorts of rules; and that ethics is about trying to make the world a better place – are both plausible. And sometimes, as we have indicated, they come into conflict with one another. These sorts of conflicts and the resulting dilemmas of choice are characteristic of ethics.

There are few ethical issues about which there is widespread agreement but many more that are subject to continuous debate. The central reason for this is that there is no generally agreed 'framework of thinking' for ethics. The common sense disagreements about ethical approach are mirrored by at least as many disagreements amongst those with an interest in ethical theory. (Indeed the distinction between rule-based thinking and consequence-based thinking is a fundamentally important distinction in ethical theory, and one we will return to from time to time.) Both within common sense or 'customary' ethics, and within ethical theory, there are a range of potential 'frameworks of thinking' competing one with another.

Here we will discuss just one potential value framework simply by way of an example (albeit an unusually influential example). This is the framework provided by the widely known four *prima facie* principles of health care ethics (Beauchamp & Childress 1994, Gillon 1990). *Prima facie* literally means 'at first sight'. In other words, at first sight – according to the proponents of this framework – all these four principles should guide our work in health care. We will set them out before briefly putting them in context:

- Respect for autonomy. This is the requirement to respect peoples' right to self-government to the extent that this right is compatible with the similar right of others.
- Beneficence. This is the requirement to produce net benefit for those on whose behalf health care workers undertake interventions.
- Non-maleficence. This is the requirement not to cause harm to those on whose behalf interventions are being undertaken.
- Concern for justice. This is understood as the requirement to act on the basis of fair adjudication between competing claims, perhaps in respect of access to resources, or with reference to rights, or in the context of legal justice.

It is possible to discern these principles or values in much writing and discussion about the ethics of health care, although they may be called different things.[1] A body of writers have suggested that these principles are owed to

---

[1] We take the terms 'principles' and 'values' to refer to overlapping ideas here. Some writers on ethics and health care – for example, Gillon (1990) – talk about 'principles'; others – for example, Downie, Tannahill & Tannahill (1996) – refer more often to 'values'. Sometimes there is little or no difference in what is actually being talked about. Gillon talks about the principles of respect for autonomy and Downie *et al.* discuss the value of respecting autonomy. But it seems reasonable to see 'values' as the generic term here, so that values might include rights, ideals, virtues etc. as well as principles.

patients or clients by health care workers by virtue of the special relationship they have with them. (Technically, this is a feature of what is referred to as 'the scope of application' of principles.) It is worth reflecting for a moment on these values and considering to what extent they reflect your own professional involvement in the field of health care. It might, perhaps, be surprising if someone working in health care didn't believe that they should try and respect autonomy, produce benefit for patients or clients and so on. This feeling is perhaps what leads an influential UK writer on the principles, Raanan Gillon, to this view:

> 'The four principles plus scope approach claims that whatever our personal philosophy, politics, religion, moral theory or life stance, we will find no difficulty in committing ourselves to four *prima facie* moral principles.... Moreover, these four principles, plus attention to their scope of application, encompass most of the moral issues that arise in health care.... What the principles plus scope approach can provide ... is a common set of moral commitments, a common moral language, and a common set of moral issues...'
>
> (Gillon 1994).

The difficulty is that, while these principles offer some help to the process of ethical assessment, by themselves they are too blunt and indiscriminate. There are degrees to which a particular intervention might meet one or other of the principles. There is also the constant possibility of conflict between the principles. This in turn leads to the likelihood of different people 'weighting' the principles differently in relation to an intervention – and thus of coming to different conclusions about what ought to have most importance in guiding our actions in a particular case.

One of the examples above will help illustrate these problems. The NHS trust no smoking policy will produce benefit for some people but not for others. It will benefit non-smokers and reduce the risks they run in relation to passive smoking. It may well benefit employees and users of the hospital who want to give up smoking, providing an impetus to do so. However, there will be a 'core' of people – committed and contented smokers – who will not benefit in any clear sense. They may want to carry on smoking (which brings them pleasure, reduction of stress and so on) and are now being restricted in doing so. Not only will the policy deny this group benefit, it may also cause them harm (by increasing their stress, prompting nicotine withdrawal symptoms and so on). For many employees and users, the policy will not disrupt their autonomy, but for the contented smokers it may do so quite dramatically – they are being 'forced' to behave in a certain way. In terms of the principle of justice, the 'entitlement' of non-smokers to 'health' (freedom from tobacco smoke) is being protected; but the 'entitlement' of smokers to continue uninterrupted with their habit (which after all is not an illegal one) is being attacked.

This leads us to the second problem related to the principles' application. There will be many cases of conflict between them. It is possible, for example, to argue that overall the no smoking policy will yield benefit. However, there is little doubt that autonomy will be disrupted for some and possibly for many. (It could be that many of the hospital trust's employees – even if they are not smokers – feel rather threatened by the restrictiveness of this measure and the surveillance it implies.) It therefore becomes clear, on this fairly superficial analysis, how there is the possibility of an activity meeting a principle only by degrees, or of its meeting one principle but coming into conflict with another.

It is clear then, that the principles are useful up to a point but cannot be applied without many other more specific value judgements being made. Many of us might intuitively feel that we ought to commit to something like these principles, but there is no reason why others should not feel that an alternative, or a more carefully specified, value framework ought to guide their health promotion practice. All that fundamentally matters is that they are prepared to articulate and defend the range of values they wish to appeal to. In that way, their ethical judgements can be open to public scrutiny and debate.

At this point, you may feel that the idea of ethically assessing health promotion work is so fraught with difficulties as not to be worth doing. There are ambiguities and complexities throughout. We return, however, to our basic contention that practice in health promotion cannot be considered 'good practice' unless its ethical acceptability is openly tested.

In the four chapters in this section there are a number of different styles in our approach to the issues being considered. Sometimes we will seem to be pursuing a specific line of enquiry through fairly close and narrow questioning. At other times, we will be generating lots of questions about an activity. These differences in style are deliberate. They indicate that the process of reflection and questioning is not a standardised one. What is important is that regardless of different styles of questioning the process of examination is careful, critical and – as far as possible – operates without unacknowledged assumptions. Our overall intention is to 'open up' value and ethical questions in health promotion (rather than to 'answer' them) in ways which support reflective professional practice.

Chapter 3
Empowerment or Control? Behavioural Counselling and Face-to-Face Education

Introduction

For many (possibly the majority) involved in the field, work with individual patients or clients forms a central part of their health promotion practice (Perkins 1999). Frequently, this 'face-to-face' work aims to encourage individuals to think about their health and consider the extent to which their current behaviour is likely to help them maintain their health; or the extent to which it puts them at risk from future disease. We may come across people who smoke, or drink heavily; others who don't appear to have a particularly healthy diet or who aren't especially physically active; and others who are sexually promiscuous. This isn't, of course, an exhaustive list of 'risky' health behaviour, but what it mentions are the kinds of things health promoters may well ask their patients or clients about. We ask about these sorts of things because we believe we know that smoking, heavy drinking, poor diet, physical inactivity and sexual promiscuity are behaviours which stand more than a fair chance of ultimately taking their toll in the form of morbidity and premature mortality.

'Face-to-face' health promotion work of this kind takes place in a large number of different settings. These include primary health care, hospitals, schools, informal youth settings, workplaces and prisons (Perkins, Simnett & Wright 1999, Tones & Tilford 1994). Thus health promoters encouraging people to think about their health behaviour – and reduce its 'risky' aspects if necessary – will include GPs, practice nurses, health visitors, district nurses, hospital medical, nursing and paramedical staff, teachers, youth workers, occupational health workers and prison medical staff. Supporting all of these are health promotion specialists, who have a history of providing training to health promoters engaged in behavioural counselling and face-to-face education – often using training models such as the Health Education Authority-sponsored 'Helping People Change' package (Health Education Authority 1993).

Behavioural counselling and face-to-face education related to health lifestyle and risk is a widespread and important health promotion activity. But why should it be included in a book about professional ethics and health promotion? If we are involved in such work, we might think of it as posing few, if any, ethical difficulties. Opportunistically raising the issue of smoking with a patient in general practice, say, appears straightforward. If he or she accepts our advice, fine. Acting on it – quitting or even simply reducing the number of cigarettes they smoke – means the risk to their health and well-being is likely to decrease substantially. If the advice isn't wanted or accepted, then the issue isn't pushed. At all times, the purpose of counselling or education is to support the patient to feel empowered in making the health choices they want. This principle of empowerment applies at any stage of the process.

But is the interpretation of this sort of activity correct? How easy is it to reconcile a wish to reduce risk with a commitment to empowerment? Can we dispute the idea of benefit almost automatically accruing from raising the issue of 'risky' behaviour and how it could be changed? What do we mean, in any case, by 'risk' and 'benefit' in this sort of context?

A case study: Vicky Bevan and the 'at risk' smoker

Vicky Bevan is a practice nurse in a large (11 000 patients shared between five partners) town centre general practice in southern England. The town, Otterbury, is a pleasant one with generally low levels of unemployment. However, it does have pockets of deprivation, one of which is a rambling and featureless council housing estate on its outskirts – Summerleas. Vicky's practice has patients from across the town, including Summerleas.

The practice falls within the boundaries of the North and Mid-Ottershire Primary Care Group (PCG). Indeed, one of the partners is Chair of the PCG, although his colleagues are to varying degrees less keen on the NHS organisational change the PCG represents (Department of Health 1998). Plans are in hand for the creation of a Primary Care Trust (PCT) based on the PCG boundaries.

It is a Friday morning and almost at the end of surgery. The last patient Vicky is due to see – a Mrs Katrina Woods – is to have blood taken for tests following a consultation with one of the GPs during which she had complained of dizzy spells. Vicky looks at Mrs Woods' records on the computer screen and automatically notes that this 30 year old woman was recalled for a repeat smear a year ago (the repeat showed no indication of abnormality); and that she is a cigarette smoker (twenty a day when the information was collected).

Vicky has never met Mrs Woods before. As she comes into the treatment room, Vicky introduces herself and from professional habit makes a mental note of Mrs Woods' appearance. She looks rather older than 30 and is less smartly dressed than some other patients the practice nurse sees from this mostly affluent town. Vicky remembers her address was a road on the Summerleas estate.

Mrs Woods seems rather agitated. Vicky assumes a nervousness about blood being drawn. She tells Mrs Woods not to worry but the patient says she is not anxious about the procedure; rather she is concerned about being on time to pick up her youngest son (nearly three) from playgroup. Vicky has a daughter of about that age so as the needle and syringes are being prepared, they chat briefly about their respective children. For Mrs Woods, the nearly three year old is the youngest of four. Her other children are five, seven and eight. She makes no mention of a partner, leading Vicky to wonder if she is a lone parent.

The blood is taken. While Vicky is sorting out labels, Mrs Woods starts to cough deeply. When the coughing has subsided, she smiles rather embarrasedly and says it's the fault of the cigarettes. The practice nurse asks how long she's been smoking and if she's ever thought about trying to quit. Mrs Woods tells her that she's been smoking since she was 15 and that while she's sometimes thought about giving up – especially since the arrival of the youngest – she's not sure she's got the 'will power'. She knows a few people who've given up for a couple of weeks and then gone back to it, probably smoking more than ever.

Vicky says that lots of people do manage to give up for good. She says this while thinking of research on the No Smoking Day initiative which showed that 16–18% of smokers claim to have given up or cut down for the Day. The research suggested that three months later, 0.5% of the quitted smokers were still not smoking (McGuire 1992). She gives Mrs Woods a leaflet and her telephone number and says that if she wants to talk more about smoking, and giving up, she would be happy to hear from her. The patient seems slightly non-plussed but thanks Vicky and leaves. A week or so later, Vicky receives a phone call from Mrs Woods saying she's been thinking more and more about the idea of quitting – could she come into the surgery and talk to her?

Starting to think about the ethics of this activity

Vicky Bevan is a conscientious practitioner, concerned to think about her work and its implications. At the moment, she is taking an open learning course in health promotion which she intends will help her accumulate further credits for her degree. The section of the course she finished a few weeks before had encouraged thinking about the ethical implications of her work. She wonders how well her face-to-face work with Mrs Woods might stand up to the process of ethical analysis.

Vicky considers that her model for working with Mrs Woods is probably based on the idea of 'helping people change' – the idea shared by many involved in the field that there is a responsibility to raise issues of health and lifestyle with patients or clients and where appropriate encourage them to think about – and if possible adopt – less 'risky' behaviours. This is a familiar approach to health promoters, and a way of working that is often taken to be a responsibility of health promoters. If we consider we have this responsibility, it seems sensible to think that it emerges from at least three connected beliefs. First, that changing behaviour will actually result in 'more health'. Second, that there is worth or value in encouraging behaviour change. Third, that we know what to do in order to help people change behaviour.

We will discuss these beliefs shortly. Before we do, however, we must ask the fundamental question: what is the *aim* of behavioural counselling and face-to-face education? This may seem an odd question to some. At first glance, it certainly does to Vicky as she starts out on the process of ethically assessing her intervention with Mrs Woods. Surely her aim is to promote the health of her patient through encouraging her to quit smoking (a 'risky' health behaviour)?

However, there are two difficulties here. The first is that while Vicky feels sure this is her own aim, she is not so certain that it is what motivates others. Behavioural counselling does not take place in a vacuum. When we engage in face-to-face health promotion activity, we are often working with just one individual (our patient or client) but there are others who have an interest in what we are doing and possibly their own reasons for encouraging or requiring us to do it (or alternatively, not to do it). These people or organisations might potentially have different aims for our activity.

Who are they and what could be their aims? In thinking about this, Vicky can clearly see that the partners in her practice will have an interest in the work she is doing. In turn, the PCG will have an interest in the practice; and the Department of Health (the government) will have an interest in the PCG as one of the 'on the ground' NHS organisations. (There may well be others who might or do have an interest in Vicky's work – for example, the local organisations concerned with monitoring health services, or her professional organisation – but she sees the partners, the PCG and government as likely to be most influential.)

What might the practice partners see the purpose of Vicky's behavioural counselling work to be? As partners in a good and responsible general practice, one of their aims will certainly be the promotion of health. But a general practice is also a business. Practices are paid to do health promotion through item of service payments (Department of Health 1996). They have an economic motivation – an economic aim – in doing (or deciding not to do) health promotion work.

Of course, there is no reason why the promotion of health and economics cannot sometimes co-exist happily together. Many people seek health and in doing so pay for it. We are thinking here of things like complementary and alternative therapies, which form a distinctive health 'market place' in which many are interested in buying and selling. It would seem just too indiscriminate to suggest that all those selling in such a 'market place' are only interested in making money and not at all in the health of their clients.

It is possible to have multiple aims for activities and there is no reason why Vicky's partners cannot be interested both in promoting health and in the practice making its way as a business. In the field of health promotion, multiple aims are likely to be the rule rather than the exception; and it is at least possible that on some occasions the aim of promoting health may be seen as less important than other aims (such as economic aims). Further, there may be occasions when the aim or aims of encouraging and doing 'health promotion' work have nothing to do with the promotion of health. This point may become clearer as we consider the potential aims the broader health service and government might have for Vicky's work.

As we have said, Otterbury and its county Ottershire are generally pleasant places in which to live. However, they are not immune from the intense competing pressures existing on health and social services at the beginning of the twenty-first century. The PCG – the organisation charged with commissioning local health care – has to take account of, and respond to, both particular local as well as national pressures.

Of the many significant local pressures, two are particularly worth mentioning here. First, Otterbury (and Ottershire) has a relatively large population of older people. This part of the country is, after all, a nice place to spend retirement. In turn, this demography makes particular demands on health services and particularly how NHS finance is spent. There is, for example, a heavily funded stroke unit at the local district hospital along with a larger than might be expected number of elderly care beds. The running of these services, and the hospital itself, is largely controlled by the consultant doctors who practice there and who are quite happy to see service provision broadly continuing as it is at the moment, and to resist any changes to the *status quo*.

On the other hand, the last few years have seen a growing concern about other population groups. Those suffering relative deprivation – which would include a large number of people living on the Summerleas estate – have received particular attention. This partly reflects renewed national interest in deprivation and inequalities in health (Benzeval, Judge & Whitehead, 1995, Secretary of State for Health 1999). It is also related to changes in the local political situation. After many years of Conservative domination of the local district and county councils, the Otterbury unitary local authority now, rather surprisingly, has a Liberal Democrat majority, determined to pursue what they see as a more radical agenda. Some of this majority membership feel that a challenge to the *status quo* of local health care provision is well overdue and are making their views known to the PCG, and to the local health authority.

The second pressure relates particularly to provision of primary health care. There are three multi-partner general practices in Otterbury, including the one for which Vicky works. In addition, there is a single-handed practice with a very small (2,500) patient list. Dr Wilson, the single-handed GP, is in his early fifties and popular with his patients. The PCG – supported by the health authority and in the context of national policy opinion concerned about single-handed practices (Department of Health 2000b) – is attempting to pressure Dr Wilson into joining with one of the other practices. Local bodies concerned with monitoring health services are sceptical about this, partly because their intelligence has shown that some patients at the other practices have felt that the GPs in these often 'just don't have the time for them'. The Chair of the PCG (who, it will be remembered, is also a partner in Vicky's practice) is lobbying to influence this perception and change practice. One of the ways he sees this as being done is through creating a more active role for the practice nurses, so enabling the doctors to concentrate on the patients they see.

How does all this relate to Vicky's intervention with Mrs Woods? These two local pressures (of course there are many more) could lead to the PCG seeing very different aims for the intervention than simply 'to promote health'. In relation to the first pressure being applied by local politicians, the PCG could see the aim of the intervention as being to contribute to a shift in the *status quo*. (Less charitably, it could be seen as aiming to contribute to keeping the radicals happy.) With regard to the second pressure – specific changes in local provision of primary health care – the aim may be viewed as helping to create a more consumer-friendly face for this provision (or again less charitably, as helping a 'take over' bid).

None of these potential alternative aims of broader health services are necessarily incompatible with the aim of promoting health. However, it is important to note their existence and, as we will shortly discuss, the impact different aims might have on an ethical assessment of Vicky's intervention.

The idea that the aim of 'health promotion' might at least sometimes be nothing to do with the promotion of health will become clearer still if we consider the potential aims a national government might have for (things such as) Vicky's health promotion intervention with Mrs Woods. It is easy, through a fairly cursory analysis of 'health headlines', to identify that health services face multiple pressures. Here is a selection taken at random:

'Delays in HIV funding attacked . . .' (Donnelly 2000).

Health authorities and voluntary organisations are expressing concern over government delay on decisions about HIV and AIDS funding allocations for the coming financial year; and about the lack of progress with the national HIV and AIDS strategy.

'Ovarian cancer drug will cost health authorities millions . . .' (Health Service Journal 2000a).

Health authorities are expected to have to find millions of pounds to fund use of the anti-cancer drug paclitaxel (Taxol) after its use with patients suffering from ovarian cancer was approved by the National Institute for Clinical Excellence.

'Poll victory for A and E campaigners . . .' (Health Service Journal 2000b).

Campaigners against the closure of a local Accident and Emergency department and the removal of this service to a larger town some miles away were heartened by significant victories in local council elections of candidates standing under the anti-closure banner.

> 'Ventilator trial inquiry finds significant errors...' (Health Service Journal 2000c).

Significant inadequacies have been found by the inquiry into a controversial ventilator trial at a Staffordshire hospital, in which 43 premature babies died or were left brain damaged.

Pressures represented by these headlines include competition for resources; the challenging of 'expert' (normally medical) power; the demand for effectiveness and efficiency from health services; and the nature of the relationship between health services and those who use them. These, of course, are only representative of some of the pressures on the NHS and, by implication, government as it tries to determine its aims in delivering health care. It follows, once more, that the idea of a single clear-sighted aim in the delivery of health care – including the delivery of health promotion – is unrealistic. It is far more likely that there will be multiple, competing aims as a direct result of competing pressures.

Is it reasonable to think of aims as being more or less ethically defensible? (Wikler 1978). Take three of the potential aims of Vicky's intervention (as understood by either herself or by others) that we have discussed above:

(1)   The aim of Vicky working with Mrs Woods is to promote (improve) her health.
(2)   The aim of Vicky working with Mrs Woods is to improve the economic performance of the practice.
(3)   The aim of Vicky working with Mrs Woods is to contribute to a change in the *status quo* of local health services.

Each of these aims carries the risk of ethical ambiguity. Consider them in reverse order. For the third aim, we might believe in the value of changing local health services and re-orienting them more to the benefit of specific disadvantaged groups. But this will depend on our point of view. What if we were an older person facing reduction in the sorts of services we are using or likely to need? For the second aim, we might be quite happy if improved economic performance was in order to improve service delivery to patients, or even to enhance staff security of employment. But what if the economic benefit received was solely for the advantage of a small number within the practice (the partners, say)? The first aim seems to carry the least ambiguity. Surely there is unequivocal value in aiming to improve the health of an individual?

This returns us to the three beliefs which we have argued are intimately connected to the putative responsibility to engage in behavioural counselling: that changing behaviour will actually result in 'more health'; that there is worth or value in encouraging behaviour change; and that we know what to do in order to help people change behaviour.

As we have already made clear, the nature of the concept of health is both elusive and contestable. (See, for example, Hare 1986, Scadding 1988, Seedhouse 2001.) More importantly in the context Vicky is considering, she knows that 'lay' concepts of health are intricate and complex (Blackburn 1991, Calnan 1987, Cornwell 1984, Herzlich 1973). This in turn may lead to ambivalent views about health behaviour and how (and whether) health should be improved.

Judgements about the meaning and desirability of health improvement are difficult to make. Vicky believes that smoking is health-harming and that the best thing Mrs Woods could do for her health would be to give up, or at least cut down. But she also knows that her view is based on her own professional and normative conceptions of health. Mrs Woods may well see things differently, even though she has asked to come and talk to Vicky about smoking. The patient may, for example, see smoking as helpful to her mental health if it allows her respite from the problems associated with raising children that she faces on a daily basis; or if she gets pleasure from the fact that cigarettes are the one luxury she allows herself (Graham 1993). At the very least, Mrs Woods is likely to feel ambivalent about smoking and its relationship with her health.

At the moment, of course, Vicky is just guessing at Mrs Woods' feelings. However, her own thoughts so far have led her to consider that there is a developing agenda of questions that need to be explored when they meet. The first of these is something like: *What does Mrs Woods think or feel is the relationship between her health needs (as she sees them) and her smoking?* Clearly this is an important question in a practical sense because if Mrs Woods thought or felt that the relationship was wholly positive, then there would be little point in working with her to quit. But it is also apparent that the question contributes to ethical exploration.

The question moves us to the second belief mentioned above: namely that there is worth or value in encouraging such change. As we have already argued, health is a value. There is dispute and ambiguity about the nature of the concept, and there is a related disagreement about the value of health in its various conceptions. The questions about Mrs Woods' beliefs and perceptions on the nature of health and smoking are, likewise, connected to further questions: *What does she value about health?; and what value does she attach to stopping smoking?*

This leads us to what we are treating as the central ethical tension within behavioural counselling and face-to-face education work: Are we attempting to empower? Or to control?

Vicky considers possible answers to the questions she has framed. On the one hand, Mrs Woods might believe that smoking is simply damaging her health, that she would have 'more health' if she was able to give up smoking, and regard this as purely valuable. In this case the goal of change assumes a *prima facie* legitimacy and the question becomes one of how to achieve it rather than whether it should be achieved at all. Alternatively Mrs Woods may be more ambivalent in her attitude towards smoking, the relationship to and the effect it has on her health (again, she might see it as positively promoting mental health). Here the value of 'more health' through quitting becomes much more contestable, simply because it is set against other understandings of the nature and value of health.

The issue is, of course, more complicated because – even simply taking Mrs Woods' perspective – 'health' is not the only value that needs to be considered. It will be one of a set that might include, say, friendship (smoking makes it easier for Mrs Woods to relax with her friends, most of whom are smokers). Such alternative values may be seen as health-related by some, but they are also important in their own right. Whether we see the issue as one of weighting different sorts of 'health-related consequences' together – friendship versus healthier lungs say – or more as a conflict between non-health and health-related values (depending upon our conception of health) there are inevitably qualitatively different, and sometimes competing, values to weigh together.

Obviously Mrs Woods' values are not the only values to consider. This chapter began by noting the assumption that appears to be made by many health professionals; their responsibility to help change the health behaviour of patients or clients. This assumption rests upon a particular conception of the value of health (as not smoking, not drinking and so on); and of the relative priority of the value. And there are of course other values, already alluded to, held by health professionals or those directing their work – economic efficiency, institutional performance, and so on. (Other key values for health promoters – such as the good of the population as a whole – are discussed more in later chapters.)

Amidst all this, Vicky considers her forthcoming exchange with Mrs Woods. It seems unlikely that Mrs Woods will straightforwardly believe that smoking is damaging to her health, that she would simply have 'more health' if she gave up and that this goal is an uncomplicated value and a first priority for her. And if these things don't apply should Vicky be engaging in this activity at all? And if (from her own motivations or as a result of pressure from others) she does, isn't she attempting to control Mrs Woods' behaviour rather than helping empower her to take the direction she wishes? [It is important, of course, to recognise that 'control' is a rather overarching term. In any intervention between a health promoter and her or his patient or client the extent to which control is being exercised will vary. Quite often, health promoters are offering gentle encouragement to patients or clients to change. We may not even consider this to constitute attempts at 'control' in the larger and more alarming senses of this word. Of course, on occasions, health promoters may exert greater levels of control through such tactics as warnings and exhortations – and possibly more. We may be inclined to view gentle persuasion as having a greater degree of ethical acceptability than strong coercion (Wikler 1978). We will return to these ambiguities later in the chapter.]

So far, Vicky has considered the possibility that Mrs Woods may not want to quit. But if Mrs Woods did in fact want to give up, Vicky feels confident she could help her. There is not much doubt in her mind about the third belief (discussed at the start of the chapter) underpinning 'helping people change'; that we know what to do in order to help people change behaviour. (Of course, this is closely connected to the first two beliefs. If we felt doubtful about our capacity to help people change then we would have a strong set of practical doubts – as well as ethical ones – about whether there is value in trying to encourage such change.)

A couple of days before seeing Mrs Woods, Vicky begins the component of her open learning course that is to do with evaluation of health promotion activity. Reading through the material, it becomes apparent to her that the issue of whether health promotion 'works' is a complex one in general and particularly so in the case of behavioural change counselling. Broadly, the material suggests to Vicky that the evidence pointing to the success of such lifestyle change in relation to smoking is slender; and what success might be possible is likely to be hard-fought (NHS Centre for Reviews and Dissemination 1998). More worrying, however, is the lack of evidence on the particular approach to change which she has been encouraged to develop and the effectiveness of which she had not previously doubted.

For Vicky, 'helping people change' in the general sense has been almost synonymous with 'Helping People Change', a training package developed in the mid-1990s (Health Education Authority 1993) and heavily promoted in the Otterbury area, as elsewhere in England. The package takes a model that attempts to explain and predict addictive behaviours (Prochaska & Diclemente 1984) – the so-called 'stages of change' model – and relates it to brief interventions that might be used by the health care professional to support 'risky' health behaviour change.

For example, a practice nurse, like Vicky, identifies a patient, like Mrs Woods, as a smoker. Although the patient might be in what is termed by the model a pre-contemplation stage, the nurse opportunistically raises the issue and provides information, possibly over several successive consultations. The pre-contemplation stage may last months or even years but eventually, at least in part because of this opportunistic contact, the patient begins actively to consider changing smoking behaviour. Again in the context of the primary health care consultation, the nurse helps the patient identify problems and benefits in changing behaviour. The patient (once more, maybe over some time) decides that benefits may outweigh problems and decides to quit smoking. The nurse helps the patient prepare for this change through identifying sources of support and helping to devise an 'action plan' for the achievement of change. The patient then changes behaviour and maintains that change, with help as required. She or he may 'relapse' at any time and return to one of the preceding stages, at which point the nurse may once more undertake interventions in relation to that stage.

Vicky attended a training course on using the 'Helping People Change' package a couple of years ago and has always found it a useful way of understanding change and planning 'interventions' since. (It was in her mind as she initially raised the issue of smoking with Mrs Woods.) Now, however, the material she is reading points to a review of the literature (Ashworth 1997) which identified little evidence comparing stage-based with non-stage-based interventions. It appears that it simply does not seem to be known whether 'Helping People Change' is any more or less effective than other ways of encouraging individual behaviour change. This brings Vicky back to the fact that in general the evidence for lifestyle change work is sketchy. One or two studies of interventions promoting individual behaviour change in the primary health care context have identified modest but arguably worthwhile results; although they have also recorded that these have often been achieved at the expense of substantial extra burdens of work (Imperial Cancer Research Fund Oxcheck Study Group 1995, Family Heart Study Group 1994).

To Vicky, none of this necessarily means that she shouldn't try and carry on helping people change. But practically it also means we may be less confident in our belief that we know what to do in order to help people change behaviour than we thought. Further, continuing to speak practically, it affects the beliefs that changing behaviour will result in 'more health' (we are simply not sure whether we have the capacity to do this here); and hence that there is value in encouraging behaviour change.

These practical doubts of course have strong implications for our earlier ethical worries. If Mrs Woods is in fact seeking to change and Vicky's role is about empowering her to do so, then the patient may be misled in her belief that change can take place. This sounds neither particularly empowering nor particularly ethical. Of course, Vicky can be honest with Mrs Woods and say she doesn't know whether she will be able to help her give up smoking, but again this doesn't sound especially empowering.

Matters become more alarming still if Mrs Woods is ambiguous about change and yet it continues to be promoted despite her apparent resistance (that is to say, if there are more strenuous attempts to control Mrs Woods' behaviour). Because here it is quite possible that no-one's goals will be achieved in the process.

Some clarifications

So far, Vicky Bevan has considered in quite a lot of detail the possible aims of behavioural counselling and face-to-face education work – those of other people or organisations, as well as her own. She has also considered what is known about the effectiveness of this kind of activity and thought about how limited knowledge in this area might impact on key beliefs about the nature and value of this sort of intervention.

This process has been helpful because it has enabled Vicky to clarify her aims and beliefs. At least as far as she is concerned, she is clear how the potential activity might match up to the value framework she has in mind for assessing the potential intervention – the 'four principles' of health care ethics. She wants to support Mrs Woods in quitting smoking if – and only if – this is what the patient herself wants. So the grounds are laid for the obligation to respect autonomy. Leading on from this, despite the worries she has about the effectiveness of smoking-related behaviour change interventions, she remains sure that if Mrs Woods wants to give up and she manages to do so, it will be beneficial to her health. The obligation to produce benefit is therefore being addressed. If Vicky is honest with Mrs Woods about the difficulties in giving up and the ambiguous evidence in this area, then the obligation to avoid harm is being considered. It is possible that there may be conflict related to the obligation to justice here, at least at other levels. Given what we know about the time and cost of behavioural change interventions, and their relative effect, it could be argued that concern for justice in the sense of fair allocation of health care resources might not be met. However, if the earlier conditions of autonomy, respect and commitment to benefit are met, then fulfilling Mrs Woods' entitlement to adequate health care may mean, at least in some respects, that the principle of justice is being considered.

But this analysis can be no more than provisional. Vicky would need to reflect further on all of these matters. Also, much depends on how Vicky's relationship with Mrs Woods develops. In particular, and based on Vicky's ethical assessment of the situation so far, there is a need: (a) to be clearer about Mrs Woods' values and priorities; (b) to be as sure as possible that Mrs Woods is making her own choices; and (c) to make sure that Vicky's purpose in working with her is to support and enable her to do so.

It is just before lunch time on Tuesday, the week following Mrs Woods' call to Vicky. The surgery is winding down after a busy morning. It is the end of May and beyond the window of Vicky's room, she sees that sunshine has enticed tourists heading for Otterbury's famous cathedral into summer clothes. There is a hesitant knock at the door.

Vicky: *Yes...?*
Mrs Woods: *Hello, am I early?*
Vicky: *No, you're fine. Please, come in and grab a seat.*
Mrs Woods: *Thanks.*
Vicky: *Are you OK for time?*
Mrs Woods: *Yes, yes, no, this is good. I don't have to pick up my youngest from the play group until half past twelve. It's nice to have a bit of time for once.*
Vicky: *It must be. I just have the one and I always seem to be rushed off my feet.*
Mrs Woods: *Well, I suppose working and everything...*
Vicky: *I suppose so. Do you work?*

Mrs Woods: *I've just started again. Part time. Office cleaning. In town. It's only evenings. Seven to nine. My mum looks after the kids. I wouldn't like Dave to do it.*

Vicky: *Dave's your...*

Mrs Woods: *My boyfriend. He moved in a couple of months ago. I mean, he's good with them and everything, don't get me wrong, but it's a lot to ask what with four of them. I mean, the older ones can play out and that, but the youngest, he's not three yet.*

Vicky: *So how are you feeling?*

Mrs Woods: *About the smoking?*

Vicky: *Well, yes – and generally.*

Mrs Woods: *I'm better than I have been. I went through a bad patch after Phil – that was my husband – left. Four children – and Daniel was only nine months. Then there was that scare with the smear. But then I met Dave and he's, you know, he's alright and now we're living together. It was him that got me to ring you up.*

Vicky: *How was that?*

Mrs Woods: *Dave doesn't smoke. Well, he used to but he gave up two or three years ago. He plays football and he said it was slowing him down. Anyway, he has this thing about me smoking. I mean, he doesn't stop me or anything – he can't, it's not his house – but, like, you know he doesn't like me doing it.*

Vicky: *And how do you feel about it?*

Mrs Woods: *What do you mean?*

Vicky: *Do you enjoy smoking?*

Mrs Woods: *I don't think I think about it really. It's just a habit. I've done it since I was at school. I mean, I suppose I ... you know, sometimes it's just nice to sit down with a cigarette. It does make me feel better sometimes. Though now I've got Dave life's better than it used to be.*

Vicky: *So if you had to say why you're here, would it be because Dave wanted you to be here, or because you wanted to be?*

Mrs Woods: *I don't know. Dave, I suppose. I mean, if the smoking's getting him down, I don't want to lose him.*

Vicky: *Why do you think it's getting him down?*

Mrs Woods: *Well, the smell and it can't be easy if you've been a smoker yourself and given up. Living with one, I mean.*

Vicky: *And presumably he's concerned about your health?*

Mrs Woods: *Yes... Oh yes, I think he is. I mean, he's a good bloke.*

Vicky: *And are you concerned about your health?*

Mrs Woods: *You mean, apart from what Dave thinks?*

Vicky: *Yes.*

Mrs Woods: *Well, I got really worried about that smear. I suppose it started to make me think about things a bit more. I mean, you know smoking's bad for you but you think, I'm young, it doesn't matter. I started when I was young, when everyone did it. Then I got into the habit and when I was having the bad time with Phil and the children being so little I just ... cigarettes became really important to me. I couldn't have given them up. I don't know if I can now. I know people who've tried and haven't managed. But the thing* *is, now I think , I'm thirty, I've got four children. I'm living with a bloke who's good to me – and the kids as well. My life's better than it has been for a while so maybe I should listen to what Dave is saying and have a go at giving up.*

Vicky: *'Should'? What do you mean?*

Mrs Woods: *No, I mean, I know that smoking isn't doing me any good.*

Vicky: *If you decided that you wanted to go ahead and give up, who would you be doing it for? For Dave, or for you?*

Mrs Woods: *Well, if I did it, I'd have to do it for me, wouldn't I?*

Vicky: *Yes. (After a pause) Do you want to do it?*

Mrs Woods: *(Another pause) Yes . . . Yes, I do.*

The practice nurse and her patient carry on talking for another twenty minutes or so but after this point, the focus of the conversation changes. Vicky becomes concerned to establish practical facts such as how many cigarettes a day Mrs Woods smokes and whether she can identify a particular pattern to her smoking – times of stress, or of socialisation, for example. She does this because she has identified that Mrs Woods wants to give up and the question becomes one of how rather than whether. In terms of the 'stages of change' model proposed above, the patient might broadly be understood as moving from contemplation to preparing to change. In order to support that move, Vicky needs to work with Mrs Woods further to identify possible barriers to change (for example, she will find it hard to do without cigarettes in some social situations where smoking is the norm). This in turn will lead to preparation of more detailed plans for change (for example, deciding to stop smoking in one of the weeks where Dave is around as much as possible for support and she is not due to go to one of her Thursday pub nights with her friends). At the end of the meeting, Vicky asks Mrs Woods to do a smoking 'diary', identifying patterns and possible flash points, which can be used for detailed planning when they meet again the following week.

Vicky is satisfied that the change in direction of her conversation with Mrs Woods can be ethically justified – at least to some degree. Before the meeting partly transcribed above, Vicky wanted to be clear about three things.

First, what did Mrs Woods think was the relationship between her health (as she sees it) and her smoking? Vicky judged that her patient saw her smoking as a behaviour with 'risky' consequences for her overall health:

Mrs Woods: *No, I mean, I know that smoking isn't doing me any good.*

Second, did Mrs Woods value the health-related goal of stopping smoking? Again, Vicky was satisfied with the response:

Mrs Woods: *Well, if I did it, I'd have to do it for me, wouldn't I?*

Vicky: *Yes. (After a pause) Do you want to do it?*

Mrs Woods: *(Another pause) Yes . . . Yes, I do.*

Vicky remains broadly happy with the provisional analysis of this activity against the 'four principles' of health care ethics. Of course, if answers had been different, the practice nurse's attitudes would equally likely have been altered. Further, there is no reason why the state of affairs that was established on this sunny Tuesday morning should remain so. Mrs Woods' views and values may change. At least part of Vicky's responsibility as a conscientious practitioner helping someone to change is to regularly check and review the views and values of those she is helping, as well as her own.

Concluding discussion: empowerment or control?

The third issue about which Vicky sought clarity must still be considered. She must be clear that her purpose in working with Mrs Woods is to support and enable the patient to make her own choices with regard to her health. Regular reviewing and clarification of one's own and others' views and values helps to address this issue. But given the very different values and expectations held by separate people involved in, or directing, health promotion, how can Vicky be sure that she is empowering and not (even if unwittingly) engaged in control of some kind?

The answer to this question, perhaps one that is difficult for practitioners to face, is that Vicky cannot be completely sure. As a committed and conscientious practitioner, she can work sensitively and supportively: she can listen, and act according to the choices and values expressed by her patient; she can be aware of the wider tensions surrounding work in this sort of area. However, none of this will completely remove the central problematics related to the idea of empowerment in the field of health promotion: First, that empowerment – contrary, perhaps, to the beliefs of many involved in the field – should not be thought of as an uncomplicated ethical value. Second, 'empowerment' and 'control' are not necessarily mutually exclusive categories. Third, whether or not an intervention is a 'controlling' one is not simply a function of the intentions of the health promoter. As we have already noted there are different degrees of 'active' control or coercion in health promotion. But it is particularly important for health promoters to recognise that some relatively subtle and low key types of influence – which may not be intentionally coercive – can embody less visible but nonetheless powerful forms of social control. In our case study, for example, however cautious and sensitive Vicky attempts to be in her style of working she is indirectly bringing to bear on her client the entire 'apparatus' of the health service and the pervasive discourses of personal responsibility for health. (For a fuller discussion of this see Duncan & Cribb (1996) or the chapters in Bunton, Nettleton & Burrows (1995).)

Health promotion theorists frequently view empowerment as representing and supporting the values of both individual freedom and of community. These values are fundamental – any attempt to limit or deny them is to deny human aspirations and therefore ultimately likely to be self-defeating. In this sense, limiting empowerment is against health itself (Dougherty 1993, Yeo 1993). Empowerment – supporting and enabling individual (and community) freedom – is, it is argued, likely to maximise chances for positive health choice (Tones 1983, 1992). Empowerment is therefore, according to some theorists, a practical strategy for getting 'more health'; and in some ways representative of the nature and value of health itself.

But all this has the feel of rhetoric. What exactly is 'empowerment'? Fielding (1996) offers two key accounts of the concept. The first is the 'process' or 'neutral' account, in which those who have power decide that appropriate others should have greater power and so 'transfer' or 'give' this power to these others. For example, in the case discussed above, others (including Vicky Bevan herself) have decided to support Mrs Woods assuming more power in relation to her health by offering information, advice and possibly more extensive resources.

The second account is the 'emancipatory' account. Here it is argued – in opposition to the first account – that empowerment is not simply 'give and take'.

'Empowerment ... is a struggle in difficult and often hostile contexts ... The point of the struggle is to realise a view of social justice and the development of the democratic way of life ...' (Fielding 1996).

This account would interpret the above example as manifestation of a 'struggle' between two or more of the parties involved – between, say, Vicky and Mrs Woods on the one hand; and those who are at the least ambivalent towards her becoming empowered (this might not be in the interests of, say, the major tobacco companies).

Both of these accounts hold difficulties for health promotion. If empowerment is 'process', it implies particular kinds of relationships; powerful individuals or organisations bestowing, through largesse, some of their own power on those who previously had none, or at least less. This does not seem to be straightforwardly 'empowering', partly because there must be questions as to who decides on 'balances of power' and how these decisions are made. Who has agreed – because this is what this account implies – that Vicky should be allowed to do this kind of work with Mrs Woods? And at what point will this work cease to be acceptable to them?

On the other hand, if empowerment is seen as 'emancipation', a 'struggle ... to realise a view of social justice', the conflict between the separate parties becomes more explicit. What is more, the conflict is essentially one of values. What is 'social justice'? Mrs Woods' views will differ from Vicky's which will differ again from, say, those of the PCG or the Department of Health and the Government (and of globally based tobacco companies).

To talk then, of behaviour change work as being about *either* empowerment or control is perhaps to try and inject artificial clarity into the situation. A more careful consideration of the idea of empowerment suggests that to some degree, at least, it involves decisions or disputes related to control: of how much power is given away; or of how much an individual should have. This is not to suggest that Vicky cannot work towards having an empowering approach in her work with Mrs Woods. We have already mentioned ways in which this might be achieved. But it does mean that questions of how much power and how much control will always be present in this kind of work.

Chapter 4
Individual or Community Interest?
Considering Teenage Pregnancy

Introduction

A central argument of this book is that the goals and methods of health promotion are open to debate. In the last chapter we explored one such debate: that is to say, the tensions between on the one hand, the 'enabling' or 'empowering'; and on the other, the 'controlling' aspects of health promotion. In this chapter we wish to develop that theme but also connect it to another, equally fundamental, tension built into the heart of health promotion. This is the tension between the good of the individual and the good of the population. Is health promotion meant to serve the individual or the community? The obvious answer is, of course, that it should serve both. But as we have seen with the idea of empowerment, there is a danger that saying this merely covers up major conflicts and ethical dilemmas.

Of course, as we discussed in Section One, there is no such single thing as 'health promotion' – it is a name for a movement which encompasses different sorts of work and different kinds of approaches to work. In part, what we are considering are tensions between the different faces of health promotion: for example, between the 'hard' public health face which tends to concentrate on population disease measures; and the 'softer' face, often represented by certain styles of health education, which tend to be more responsive to individual concerns. It is important however, to stress that health promoters cannot simply make a global choice between 'individual' and 'community'; or between 'soft' and 'hard'. These tensions are built into all of the small choices that health promoters make; and they create real dilemmas because there are valuable things pulling in conflicting directions.

In this chapter, we will use the general focus of sexual health promotion, and more specifically issues around teenage pregnancy, to explore these ethical tensions. Is teenage pregnancy a problem at all? Why should it be a concern of health promoters? Is it a problem for society at large? Or is it a problem solely for those individual young people experiencing teenage pregnancy? How far should health promoters be guided by public perspectives, or by their own personal ones? If you are a health promoter facilitating local 'teenage pregnancy' service development, what kinds of issues do you face, and how might you think about them? These are some of the questions prompting the discussions in this chapter. To begin with, we will introduce some of the general themes of our discussion: the relationships between sex and ethics; between individuals and communities; and the nature of teenage pregnancy. In the second part of the chapter, we will use the Department of Health's recent 'Guidance on Tackling Teenage Pregnancy' (Department of Health 2000a) as the framework to develop our discussion.

Introducing the themes

Sex and ethics

It is impossible to discuss sex and ethics without getting 'hijacked' by other value questions and concerns. We begin by acknowledging this fact. Indeed, it is perhaps not strictly 'hijacking' at all, because questions about social and personal values are closely tied up with sex and sexuality.

Sometimes, the word 'morality' is almost equated with sexual morality. If someone is accused of 'immoral conduct', the assumption many people will make is that they are suspected of some sexual misdemeanour; and not, for example, that they have been cruel to their employees. Sex and ethics are closely linked. In many respects this makes good sense. After all, like 'life and death', sex is a basic feature of human experience, a biological given and a crucial part of social and cultural life. Some of the most important and socially divisive ethical debates we face – for example, around contraception and abortion – are connected with these themes. (Consider, for example, the nature of arguments about abortion in Dworkin (1995).) However, there is often something strange going on in the equating of sex with 'morality'. The name of 'morality' can be invoked simply to gesture towards a taboo, or to condemn a person or practice. It is often applied not merely to suggest that something is wrong, but – as it were – to 'make' it wrong, bad, rotten, 'unnatural', inhuman. Something of this sort is going on when some people describe homosexuality as immoral. They are seeking to put it 'beyond the pale' – to shun and condemn it. They are not, it seems to us, making a point about ethics. Rather, they are trying to assert that their values are not values at all, but instead are objective facts. And they are doing so without reasoned explanation or justification.

It is important that we explain these comments further. They leave us open to the following charge: 'You find homosexuality acceptable but other people do not. You are criticising people for being prejudiced but in so doing you are merely displaying your own prejudices.' We hope we are not guilty in this respect. We are not saying that someone cannot advance ethical arguments against homosexuality or homosexual lifestyles. Quite the opposite. We are prepared to consider such arguments. (Roger Scruton has advanced arguments of this sort in his book, Sexual Desire: A Moral Philosophy of the Erotic (1986).) Once arguments are in the public domain they can be considered and debated. We are not trying to rule out the possibility of criticism of homosexuality, or of any other aspect of sexual life. We are simply making a distinction between considered ethical debate and 'blind' taboos. It is important to do this because sexuality is an area where taboos, unreflective prejudices and moralism exercise a lot of power.

Very powerful social norms exist which can serve to 'validate' or 'invalidate' sexual behaviours. These norms shape our personal and cultural identities in a variety of ways; we are all involved in these processes of normalisation and stigmatisation. Thus our motivations and evaluations are inextricably caught up in a web of overlapping and competing sexual 'norms'. Moreover, sexuality is an area where there are generally strong motivating forces. It is no accident that we use the word 'lust' to describe not only specifically sexual desire; but also any particularly strong or passionate desire. Sexual desire is often seen as emblematic of the tension between on the one hand the need we generally have socially to regulate and control our behaviour; and on the other, to pursue our atavistic passions. There are a host of social and psychological mechanisms designed to 'civilise' and manage sexual desire – yet TV chat shows are full of stories of individuals who are struggling to manage their sexuality!

These facts have implications for anyone embarking on a consideration of sex and ethics. First, they remind us that there are pressures and motivations associated with sex which will have to be taken into account. No-one can simply 'legislate' for sexuality and expect everyone else to jump accordingly. Second, they mean that we should always subject statements about sexual ethics to particular scrutiny. Do they really stem from some kind of ethical reflection? Or are they merely 'dressed up' prejudices? As we shall see, moralism of this latter kind plays a substantial role in the debates about teenage pregnancy.

These considerations make some people inclined to dismiss all discussion of sexual ethics. They lump together all judgements about sexual ethics – simply because they are about sex – as if they must be blind prejudices. Thus, reasoned discussion in this area is not possible. This, however, is an overreaction which, if we were to accept it, would exclude a fundamental area of human experience from ethical examination. After all, we can have ethical debates about playing tennis: are there any circumstances in which it is acceptable to cheat?; is it acceptable to question line calls?; does playing tennis for money necessarily have a corrupting effect on the culture of the game? Although these are not necessarily important questions (to most of us), they are ethical questions. It would seem very odd to suppose that you could consider and debate questions of 'tennis ethics', but not questions of sexual ethics.

The tensions between the individual and the community

Our principal theme for this chapter is, as we have said, the potential tensions between the needs of the individual; and those of the community. It might be worth sketching out some of these tensions. They are not mysterious or strange things – we live with them all the time. The relationship between the individual and the family (a very small community) demonstrates many of the issues in microcosm.

When making choices, families have to take into account the interests of their constituent members. It is important to stress that these interests do not neces-sarily conflict. Everyone in a family may have an equal interest in taking a holiday in the sun or in moving to a more comfortable house. Everyone may strongly endorse these choices and show their appreciation of them. However, as we all know, it is not always like this. Day-to-day family life is a continuous process of negotiation, compromise and sacrifice. Conflicts of interest are weighed up and decisions often produce 'winners' and 'losers'. Within some close-knit families these tensions may not be referred to as 'conflicts'; the need to forge peaceable resolutions to them, and to serve the collective good of the family, would make this kind of language unattractive. By contrast, here we are deliberately stressing the underlying tensions rather than their resolution.

The following are a few familiar examples of more or less important conflicts of interests within families:

One family member has a serious illness which 'requires' other family members to adapt their living arrangements, lifestyle, career, eating and sleeping patterns and so on. This may be done willingly, but it is quite possible – and understandable – that some family members may experience a strong tension between these demands and other things which they regard as important, including their own health.

The family is invited to a rare weekend reunion with members of the extended family in a distant city. Most members want to go, but one wants them to stay at home to support him in some activity that 'clashes' with the reunion.

Most of the family members like to have the living room dimly lit with a few table lamps, but one prefers to have bright light and wishes to keep the main light on whenever they are in the room.

The family faithfully follows a religious tradition and observes its practices, except for one member who wants the freedom to engage in practices that are regarded as unacceptable and wrong by the others.

Obviously it would be possible to extend and expand these four examples inde-finitely. The tensions they describe are commonplace. The examples may, of course, be different in importance. They are also different in kind. Let us call them, by way of summary, conflicts of benefits, conflicts of wants and conflicts of values. (We do not wish to imply that these ideas are exclusive, as will become clear.) The first example is an example of conflict of benefits. We are assuming that the family members are happy to choose their caring role and that it is consistent with their values. Nonetheless, they are 'missing out' on things which they would have otherwise had. The second and third examples might also be cases of benefit conflict, although they are expressed here primarily as conflicts of wants (or choice). The extent to which individuals might be harmed by having their preferences overridden is unclear and will vary from case to case. The fourth example is clearly a conflict of values; but it can also be seen as a conflict of wants and most probably also as a conflict of benefits – that is to say, the family is likely to regard the forbidden practices as intrinsically harmful, although the 'maverick' individual may take the same view about the religious practices and teachings followed by the rest. An overarching dimension of all the examples is that of the distribution of power in the family: how are decisions made; who participates; and whose voices count the most?

All the above examples at the microcosmic level of the family as community, can be replaced with similar kinds of examples existing at societal level. It is unreasonable to expect individuals to live together in the same community – whether this is understood as a family or in a much broader sense – without experiencing conflicts of interest relating to benefits, wants and values. Of course the tensions at a societal level are likely to be even more complex and, typically, there will not be the same assumptions about cohesiveness and the importance of the collective good which pertains in some close-knit families or social groups. At the population level it is more likely that individuals will see themselves as part of an abstract mass of separate individuals and families. Some people may take the idea of the societal collective good seriously – but many others will not.

Before turning to the example of teenage pregnancy in order to explore these tensions between the needs and wishes of the individual and those of the community in more depth, we will briefly indicate how they impact upon health promotion more generally.

There are some relatively clear examples of benefits conflict between the individual and the community in relation to health promotion. Population health may be benefited, say, by a particular form of vaccination although a small number of individuals may suffer as a result. Again, fluoridation of water supplies has some health benefits for the majority, but also has some other health-related costs to a small minority. Or some judgements about the allocation of resources for health promotion (for example, the decision to target a particular campaign at a particular group) will inevitably benefit some more than others.

There are also many examples of actual and potential conflicts of choice and values. There is, say, a majority preference for banning smoking in a hospital trust, although some users and employees are smokers and would prefer to be able freely to continue with their habit. Again, education about drug use might be made compulsory in a school through popular parental consent, but some parents would prefer it not to be included in the curriculum. Finally, a young people's advisory service offers information about contraception even though some think it wrong for young people (or indeed anyone else) to use contraception.

Together, these examples demonstrate one of the reasons why the analogy with families is simplistic. A society is made up from a number of groups and communities – it is not simply the aggregation of many separate individuals. There are times, then, when we also have to think of the relationships that exist between particular individual communities and the broader society. So, to take the last example above, the 'some' we refer to might be individual people; but it might also be certain religious communities who collectively wish to find expression for their values and way of life inside the wider society.

What is wrong with teenage pregnancy?

Sexual health promoters faced with the task of 'doing something' about teenage pregnancy need to ask themselves a series of questions: Is teenage pregnancy a problem?; if so, why, when and for whom is it a problem? What sorts of things can and should be done about it? What role is there for health promotion? Who has responsibility for bringing about change? How should we evaluate any change that occurs? (This list of questions is not intended to be exhaustive.)

We wish to stress the importance of the first question in this list – is teenage pregnancy a problem? – and spend a little time discussing it. As we have already argued, a fundamental ethical responsibility of health promoters is critically to scrutinise what they have been asked to do. Simply because someone in authority says, 'We need to do something about X', it does not follow that this is true. Health promoters have to work with other professionals, specific clients and the public and in so doing they effectively 'translate' policy into practice. Unless they critically scrutinise policy they may simply translate unfair and ineffective policy into unfair and ineffective practice. If they bring a critical eye to bear on their work they may, at least, be able to moderate some of these effects through the way they interpret and apply policy in practice.

So, what, if anything, is wrong with teenage pregnancy? If we stop and reflect on this question it soon becomes obvious that there are no easy answers. The expression 'teenage pregnancy' seems to cover so many different kinds of cases. Because of this, becoming pregnant can, for teenagers, as with any other age group, be regarded either as a problem, or as something wholly positive, to be celebrated (or as something in between these two positions). Of course, pregnancy inevitably carries certain risks and there is a tendency within modern societies to medicalise it (Donnison 1988). From this point of view pregnancy is generally viewed as a 'risky condition' (Enkin, Keirse & Chalmers 1989). Medicalisation is certainly an important dimension of the sexual health agenda, but again this applies to all women. It does not wholly account for the problematisation of teenage pregnancy. For an explanation of this, we need to look at popular discourse and the moralism built into it.

To elements of the media and sections of the public imagination, the expression 'teenage pregnancy' represents a multitude of sins. It picks out a decline in moral standards. In particular, it points to the uncontrolled sexual behaviour of young people – schoolgirls robbed of their childhood and life prospects, who are bringing disadvantaged children into the world for other people to look after. Of course, in reality every case is different. Even if we were to take these censuring attitudes seriously, they do not always necessarily apply; a pregnant teenager can be a 19 year-old married woman who planned her pregnancy and did not engage in sex before marriage for religious reasons. As a matter of fact, if we were to pick a pregnant teenager (in England) at random, we are 12 times more likely to find someone over, rather than under, the age of 16 (SEU, 1999). Any equating of teenage pregnancy with images of young schoolgirls is misleading from an objective, statistical viewpoint.

These reflections suggest a number of provisional responses to the question of what is wrong with teenage pregnancy. First, in many respects it is a problem at the global, societal level; it is not necessarily a difficulty for individual teenagers who become pregnant (although of course it sometimes may be so). Second, it is partly a 'socially constructed' problem; that is to say, it is in some measure a problem because teenage pregnancy symbolises broader concerns and anxieties about the nature and direction of modern society. Third, health promoters working on teenage pregnancy must take this into account and look beyond these social constructions to individual situations. If we have to generalise it is probably wisest to say that teenage pregnancy is not a problem at all. There is nothing wrong with teenage pregnancy *per se*. It is an indirect label for a whole cluster of issues which require separate consideration. These include under-age sex, unintended pregnancy, unwanted pregnancy, sex outside stable relationships, abortion, single parenthood, unwaged parenthood and unmarried motherhood. These things are all suggested by the idea of teenage pregnancy but none of them – whatever we think about them – should be equated with it.

Linda Gordon explains that teenage pregnancy is effective as a symbol 'precisely because it can express so many different laments abut society' (Gordon 1997). She encourages us to see the focus on teenage pregnancy as a 'discourse'; that is, a set of languages and 'stories' which make up our society's understanding of itself. These stories are bound up with attitudes of moralism and censure; and systematically blend together the rather different issues listed above and the experiences of different individuals. She asks us to see the discourse of teenage pregnancy in the context of state control of sexual immorality and as a political issue which differentially affects people who are poor, including, for that reason, certain minority ethnic groups. With all this in mind, she asks us to look at the issues not moralistically, or prejudicially, but ethically:

'Experts as much as citizens have a responsibility to address explicitly what is wrong with teenage pregnancy and teenage and out-of-wedlock childbearing, ethically as well as medically and economically, in the context of the actual class and racial situations of the teenagers...' (Gordon 1997).

Gordon is drawing our attention to the very different sets of life circumstances in which people form their preferences and make their choices. Any judgements we make about teenage pregnancy must be sensitive to these differences. This does not prevent us from making ethical judgements, but it does mean that we should avoid blanket judgements – still more, blanket moralisations.

At this point it might be argued that teenage pregnancy is a bad example for a discussion on the ethics of sexual health promotion. If it is not a single issue but a whole cluster of issues: and if it is a symbol for social judgement and moralisation; would it not be better to choose another, less contentious, example? Although it does raise a complex set of issues (and it would be nice if life were simpler) we would suggest that this complexity is in fact characteristic of sexual health promotion. To demonstrate this, consider the cluster of difficult issues that surround work on HIV prevention: attitudes towards homosexuality, heterosexual and homosexual promiscuity, sex industry workers and those who use their services, the conceptualisation by some that HIV/AIDS are representative of some kind of God-given judgement; these are just some of the issues that might be encountered in discussion on this topic. We suggest that difficulties and complexities emerge in relation to any topic related to the area of sexual health promotion. In general, it is an area where a wide range of medical and social issues interconnect; and where value judgements and social pressures are constantly present.

However, there is also another reason why we have chosen the compound category of teenage pregnancy as an example of an area in which tensions between the good of the individual and that of the population are exposed through health promotion work. Teenage pregnancy is a 'real world' category. By this we mean that policies and strategies are actually developed, and people are in reality employed, to 'tackle' teenage pregnancy. For the remainder of the chapter we will frame our discussion within this more practical point of view. We will reflect further on some of the themes we have already introduced, and some other theoretical themes, but we will also try to bring the discussion down to earth, because this is how many people have to deal with it in practice; as real work that they are required to do.

Tackling teenage pregnancy

The Department of Health's Teenage Pregnancy Unit 'has been set up to oversee the Government's action plan for teenage pregnancy and co-ordinate action required at a national level' (Department of Health 2000a). The plan also requires action at a local level with the appointment of co-ordinators to act as:

> 'The local champion for action and services to prevent teenage pregnancy and support teenage parents, and lead the process of local co-ordination...'
> (Department of Health 2000a).

Imagine you have been appointed to a post something like the one envisaged here – one where the purpose is to lead, or support, a local response to teenage pregnancy. From the outset, you will be confronted with three broad 'layers' of ethical issues. Even if you do not feel in a position to resolve any of them, you will have to find a way in which they can be managed.

The first layer relates to substantive ethical issues about sexual behaviour or pregnancy. The second relates to the legitimacy of public policy or health promotion activities. The third relates to 'professional practice'.

For example, you may well be asked to work on the issue of contraception for under-16 year olds. You will have some view of the ethical acceptability of contraception for under-16s and you will be aware that there are views other than yours (the first layer). Suppose you are asked to help support increased access to contraception for this age group. You may, for example, be liaising with community pharmacists, headteachers and school nurses to ensure that there is relatively easy access to emergency contraception (the 'morning after pill'). In these circumstances, therefore, you will have to make a judgement about the legitimacy of a health promotion intervention. Is it right for the state, or for professionals, to enable under-16s to access contraceptives (of whatever sort) when many people object to it? (the second layer). Given these debates, how should you proceed? Should you take a strong line in support of the policy or should you implement it cautiously? Would it be sensible to try and find ways of accommodating the views of people who object or should you 'ignore' these voices? (the third layer). These three layers interlink but they also need to be considered separately.

In what follows we will set out a little more of the background to the current teenage pregnancy initiative and explore further some of the issues raised in these 'layers of ethics', particularly the latter two. These discussions will draw us back to the overarching theme of the tension between the good of the individual and that of the community or population.

The Teenage Pregnancy Action Plan in summary

The Government's action plan was first introduced as part of a very thorough and well researched report produced by the Social Exclusion Unit (SEU 1999). Anyone who wishes to consider in depth the plan, and the background to it, should refer to this report as we cannot do it justice here.

The report stresses that the UK has high teenage conception and birth rates compared to the rest of Western Europe; in England alone over 15 000 teenagers under 18 have an abortion each year. It then sets out some of the reasons why these statistics matter, some possible explanations for them and steps that might be taken to address them. We will come back to why it matters and possible explanations later. Here we will simply include the action plan summary. It sets out the need for:

- 'A national campaign, involving Government, media, voluntary sector and others to improve understanding and change behaviour.
- 'Joined-up action with new mechanisms to co-ordinate action at both national and local levels and ensure that the strategy is on track.
- 'Better prevention of the causes of teenage pregnancy, including better education in and out of school, access to contraception, and targeting of at-risk groups, with a new focus on reaching young men, who are half of the solution, yet who have often been overlooked in past attempts to tackle the issue.
- 'Better support for pregnant teenagers and teenage parents, with a new focus on returning to education with child care to help, working to a position where no under 18 lone parent is put in a lone tenancy, and pilots around the country providing intensive support for parent and child...' (SEU 1999).

Of course this is only an outline – the plan will evolve and be revised as it is interpreted and implemented over time. However, this is enough to see the scope and complexity of the issues involved. As a local co-ordinator faced with this broad agenda you will hardly know where to begin! However, some things are clear. You will obviously have to work with different sectors and agencies including schools, health services and housing agencies. Collectively you will have to employ different kinds of strategies – educational, social and structural. You will need to find ways of reconciling and balancing 'preventive' and 'supportive' goals, each of which have rather different orientations. In doing so, you will have to try to achieve a measure of coherence and co-ordination both locally and nationally.

Implementing and co-ordinating value judgements

Although it is unlikely to appear on the job description or person specification for the post of co-ordinator, you will have to be good at what we refer to as 'implementing and co-ordinating value judgements'. (Indeed any reflective health promoter involved in the kind of work set out by the action plan needs a strong awareness of the value judgements emerging from and relating to it.) As we have seen, all health promotion policies necessarily rest on value judgements. Judgements relate to: first, the way in which the 'problem' is defined; second, what are taken to be indicators of 'success' in dealing with it; and third, why some strategies are favoured over others. If you are implementing a set of policies which cohere with a national action plan you will, at least to some degree, be working within the 'value parameters' of the plan. There may be some scope for difference of emphases, for responding to local agendas and needs, or even for challenging aspects of the plan – but the broad framework is set. As we mentioned earlier the very least you must do in order to be an informed and reflective practitioner, is to subject the value judgements about 'problem definition', 'success' and 'strategy' to critical scrutiny.

If we examine the rationale for the national action plan more closely, we see that it encompasses multiple problems (for example, limited access to education or to services providing contraception): multiple criteria of success (such as improving understanding and changing behaviour); and multiple strategies (for example, campaigns, support, targeting of particular 'at risk' groups). The value framework is thus provided partly by the balance and emphases within these accounts of problems, success criteria and strategies for action.

In particular, we need to pay attention to how success is specified in the overall goals. This provides perhaps the sharpest indication of what the teenage pregnancy action plan is 'for'. (It is not unusual for health promotion policy documents to be written in a way that embraces a broad range of needs and concerns but then to be tied to targets which place strong emphasis only on a sub-set of these concerns.) The goals of the action plan are specified in the following way:

'The Government's goals for teenage pregnancy are to:

- 'Halve the rate of conceptions among under 18 year olds in England by 2010; and set a firmly established downward trend in conception rates for under 16s by 2010.
- 'Achieve a reduction in the risk of long term social exclusion for teenage parents and their children. This will be measured using the increase in sustained participation by teenage parents in education, employment or training as a key indicator . . .' (Department of Health 2000a).

These joint goals reflect the underlying analysis that teenage pregnancy is both a cause, and a consequence, of social exclusion. Young people who are excluded or alienated from other life opportunities 'see no reason not to get pregnant . . .'. In turn they are more likely to 'live in poverty and unemployment and be trapped in it through lack of education, child care and encouragement . . .' (Department of Health 2000a).

The first goal is apparently based on the straightforward assumption that teenage pregnancy is a 'bad thing' so that less of it will necessarily be a good thing. Even the second goal, which is couched as a project of 'support' and which, arguably, is more accepting of teenage pregnancy, is also presented, according to the logic of the report as long term prevention. The tenor of the analysis summarised above is that pregnancy is a 'harm' which afflicts some teenagers. (This tone runs through much of the rest of the Social Exclusion Unit's report, although to be fair, there are also other voices present.) 'Risk factors' for teenage pregnancy are listed – poverty, being in care, being a child of a teenage mother, educational problems, exclusion post-16, sexual abuse, mental health problems, and crime. The compound effects of these 'multiple risk factors' are analysed. There is a sense that, through this epidemiological approach, teenage pregnancy is being treated much as a preventable disease.

According to the report, it seems that, at best, teenage pregnancy is something which young women 'drift into' because of otherwise unfulfilled and problematic lives. Does this mean that it cannot be seen as a positive choice, as an expression of personal autonomy, as a valid means of becoming fulfilled rather than simply as a barrier to fulfilment? There is a danger that the value framework built into the overall goals precludes these alternative perceptions. It may be that, considered in general, teenage pregnancy is a 'harm' that ought to be reduced. However, for some individuals, this 'diagnosis' is likely to be wrong. (In this regard, the analogy with disease we have suggested the report might be drawing would clearly be misleading.) As someone who is 'tackling' teenage pregnancy, how can you do justice to the general picture, but also to the specific needs and perceptions of individuals? To a large extent, this will obviously depend upon which combination of strategies are deployed in practice, and what 'messages' they convey. Before turning to that, however, it is worth asking what else might be contained in the value framework of the national plan; and what other value tensions might it contain?

Why does it matter to me?

The report contains a section entitled 'Why it matters'. However, as a local worker you will have to ask, 'Why does it matter to *me*?' In other words, which of the ways the problem is defined do I accept and which do I think are more important? Unless these questions are asked, there is the risk that you will simply be implementing work strongly infused with the value judgements of others. If this is the case, you will not be able to do your job of 'championing' action and services – you will lack both the motivation and the vision because the values driving the work are not your own (or at least have not been subject to a process through which you have worked out their acceptability or your capacity to compromise on them).

The 'harms' mentioned in the report can be divided roughly into harms to teenage parents: harms to their children; and harms to society. We will summarise some of these below. Which of these things matter to you and which do you think are the most important?

In terms of harms to teenage parents. Someone could argue – plausibly – that, with hindsight, most young women wish they had waited to become pregnant and would prefer to have had a planned pregnancy (for some even sex itself is forced or unwanted). Teenage parents tend to remain poor and are disproportionately likely to suffer relationship breakdown and social exclusion.

Considering harms to the children of teenage parents. The death rate for babies of teenage mothers is 60% higher than for babies of older women. They are more likely to have low birth weights, childhood accidents and be subjected to hospital admission. In the longer term, they are more likely to experience family break-ups and are at increased risk of living in poor housing and being badly nourished.

In terms of harms to society. Teenage pregnancy contributes to, and perpe-tuates, the social exclusion of significant numbers of poor young people. Teenage pregnancy 'costs' society through its impact on services and benefits. It also arguably has a longer-term 'cost' through its preventing some people, in eco-nomic as well as other senses, from contributing to society according to their full potential.

Even this short list indicates the complex of personal, medical, social and economic 'harms' which need balancing and co-ordinating. Here, however, we will focus on just one crucially important issue for health promotion ethics. In working on the issue of teenage pregnancy, do I want to promote personal autonomy and informed choice (of 'at risk' young people, pregnant teenagers and teenage parents); or do I want to promote some specific ends (that is to say, to prevent some at least of the 'harms' listed above)?

Once again, it is possible to see how the empowerment-control tension debated in Chapter Three overlaps with the individual-community tension, and how crucial they are. At first sight it might seem that the 'informed choice' and the 'harm prevention' model support one another. If teenagers are provided with the information and personal and social resources to enable them to make choices about sexual behaviour, they will choose not to become pregnant and so various harms will be prevented. (Many would emphasise the social resources here – the need to change the economic circumstances and 'opportunity set' available to socially excluded young people.) This may well be true to some degree at least (and it would be possible to collect empirical evidence to explore the relationship between circumstances and choices). However, it is again essential to see that these models – 'informed choice' and 'harm prevention' – conflict in principle (as well as in their practical application and outcome). According to the former model, teenagers choosing to become pregnant and have babies could be an indicator of success (providing they were sufficiently informed and autonomous and so *had made the choice*); according to the latter, teenage pregnancy would necessarily be an indicator of failure because of the various other medical and social harms which would ensue. How do you believe teenage pregnancy should be viewed, and why?

To crystallise the issues lying behind the choices you might make with regard to this question, here are brief accounts of the views of three people who have had time to think about the subject before – Marion, Gita and Genevieve. There are, of course, many other possible views, some of which are a combination of ones adopted by our 'respondents'. It is likely that you may agree partly with one of them on some issues but with another on different issues.

Marion's view

I think if people are old enough to have sex and want to, they should be allowed to have it. Lets not forget people are marrying later and also becoming 'biologically mature' at a young age – we cannot expect them to abstain from sex for the 15 years between! We need to address issues of poverty and disadvantage first. But both boys and girls also need to have a lot of sex education because they need to be able to resist pressure to have sex and they shouldn't have unprotected sex unless they are aware of the risks of infection and pregnancy. Health educators need to give young people choices and hope they use them wisely, but they shouldn't try to stop them having sex because its their choice and anyway you can't stop them. If teenagers become pregnant, they need to be treated like anyone else. A lot of them will be happy to be pregnant and will be good mothers and fathers. Both parents need to be supported to do what is a difficult job for anyone and should not be judged and stigmatised by other people.

Gita's view

I agree with Marion about some things but I think what she says about sexuality mainly applies to older teenagers. I don't think that people under about 16 are mature enough to handle the pressures and responsibilities that go with being sexually active. That's why we have the law to protect them until they are older. On the whole that's a good thing. Just because you're physically capable of having babies (or having abortions) does not mean you are capable in other ways. Also, as a society we have to make sure that babies are going to be OK and properly looked after. So you can't exactly stop teenagers from having sex, but you can make it less likely by putting social pressure on them as well as by educating them. We have to think of the overall picture – all of the costs of teenage pregnancy. If that means actively encouraging teenagers (whatever their age) not to have children then that's a small price. After all we know that most of those who do get pregnant wish they had planned more carefully.

Genevieve's view

I think Marion misses the point completely, and Gita means well but doesn't really get it. It's not just about whether teenagers should be allowed sexual freedom or whether we should try to prevent the social costs of teenage pregnancy. The point is that we want our young people to have full lives, worthwhile lives, and lives of integrity. Of course social disadvantage needs tackling but we also have to think about what sorts of lives people should live. We need to help young people understand that sexual behaviour and parenthood are only really fulfilling as part of stable committed relationships. Outside such relationships we should encourage sexual abstinence. We need to restore the importance of family relationships and this will help to build a more ethical society and happier lives. This may call for social pressures and for education, but these things should not just be aimed at reducing medical harms or economic costs etc. They should be aimed at ethical change and towards an enriched society for everyone.

A local co-ordinator is likely to find themselves in meetings with people who have this range of views and others beyond. Some will have very strong views, for example, on contraception and abortion. How would you decide how to respond to them and how much notice to take of what they say? If we look at the different sorts of harms listed above along with the views of Marion, Gita and Genevieve we can see that the examples of 'family conflicts' cited earlier in the chapter are comparatively simple. Teenage pregnancy faces health promoters with a mass of conflicts of benefits, choice and values. Interests have to be weighed together and not everyone's view can be taken into account equally. Teenage pregnancy services and education would look very different if they were planned according to the views of a Marion, Gita or Genevieve. Who should you listen to?

Avoiding the disputes – views, facts and values

Perhaps we can side-step these difficult questions. After all, why should health promoters simply respond to peoples' 'views'? Clearly there is a need to treat people with respect and to listen to what they say; however, just because someone has a 'view', it doesn't mean we should build it into our planning. Some people may think the moon is made of cheese but this does not mean that NASA should send a cheese expert as the next astronaut! More seriously, some people believe that rock crystals can heal but this does not mean that the local health trust should add them to their hospital formularies. Surely we should look at the evidence for these beliefs? What are the facts, or what is the best knowledge we have available? This will provide us with a neutral basis to resolve disputes.

This quite reasonable position is what lies in part behind the drive towards evidence-based health care. We will look at the issues raised by this drive more thoroughly in the following two chapters. Here we are merely asking if it might help us to resolve the disputes between the range of different views expressed in relation to teenage pregnancy. Could we not simply assemble the facts to the best of our ability and let the outcome decide our policies? The short answer, we would argue, is no.

Of course, investigating the evidence and collecting the statistics is important and useful. This sort of research helps to settle some factual questions but it cannot settle ethical questions. Empirical investigation of this sort can help us understand the nature and scale of 'the problem'. It can also help us look for explanations as to why teenage pregnancy is more common in some countries, or some groups; or to evaluate the effectiveness of different interventions (research about all these things is marshalled in the Social Exclusion Unit's report). Of course, some of the research evidence will be ambiguous or open to conflicting interpretation. For example, most people would agree that earlier (appropriate) sex education delays, rather than advances, the age at which people start having sex, but some believe the opposite. Nonetheless, despite the inevitable disagreements which accompany all scientific and social research, trying to get at 'the facts' is helpful.

What is more, this research has critical *relevance* to the questions of value which permeate debates on teenage pregnancy. All ethical claims about this (or any other) issue have built into them claims or assumptions about facts which are open to research. If I say that I am against supplying under-16s with contraception services because this will encourage under age sexual activity, then research which shows that in fact this does or does not happen is most relevant. If research shows that this does not happen – and if I accept this evidence – I will have to revise my view in some way. I will need either to drop my objection, or point to some other negative consequence, or decide that I am simply against it 'in principle'. (And, in this case, many others may, quite reasonably, cease to take my objections quite as seriously.) So facts are relevant to value judgements but, as this example indicates, they do not settle value disputes on their own.

However, there may still be some hope for avoidance tactics. Perhaps we cannot avoid the value disputes in our conversations, but it might still be possible to ignore some of them by arguing that public policy generally, and health promotion specifically, should strive to be as neutral as possible. Although we will have to acknowledge the existence of a range of value positions these should not form the basis for health promotion. This should be based, as far as possible, on objective measures of harms, benefits and effectiveness. To many people this will seem a plausible position. It is a position which is often implicit in an epidemiological approach to health promotion. This plausibility is strengthened by a widespread liberal ideology in some societies – including that of the UK, to which the teenage pregnancy action plan applies – to the effect that individuals should be left alone to choose their own values. Neither the government nor government agencies or professionals should try to promote values. They should merely support individuals in living the lives they choose to live. Both the scientific influence and the liberal ideological influence on health promotion push in the direction of professional neutrality.

However, the drive for neutrality cannot go very far in practice. In the end, governments and professionals cannot be completely neutral. How, for example, can a government be neutral between those people who believe pregnant women should be allowed easy access to abortions and those who consider abortion to be 'murder'? If it makes abortion illegal, then it is dismissing the values of people in favour of 'a woman's right to choose'. If it allows abortion, under certain circumstances, it is dismissing the values of those who see abortion as unjustified killing. The government is – in the eyes of this group – allowing murders to take place. It is no good to say that if choice is allowed, both sets of values can be respected. Anti-abortionists are not merely saying that they would not choose abortions in their own lives; they are saying that this choice should not be permitted. In practice, there is no way to be neutral between these two value sets.

Although this is a dramatic example, the same is essentially true in many other cases. Public policies and health promotion practices will necessarily reflect certain value positions more than others. Health promoters may take on the guise of neutrality, but this will only have the effect of obscuring the values they serve.

To illustrate this, ask yourself how you would work with the 'model' health promoter described below – Mr T – the 'technician':

Mr T

> Mr T is wary of making value judgements. As a technician, he sees it as his job to proceed as if teenage pregnancy was an objective harm which we need to prevent. His activity is pure 'preventive medicine'. He confines his attention to those harms and benefits which he sees as objectively measurable (for example, death rates, birth weights, financial costs). Whatever techniques work to 'solve' the problem should be considered. He is, in fact, purposefully agnostic about the ethical arguments for and against under age sex, contraception or abortion. Similarly arguments which advocate ideals of behaviour, or relationships, or family life as representing better, more fulfilled lives, leave him cold. His position is, 'Anything goes, so long as it works'. If an educational package promoting sexual abstinence was found to be extremely effective at meeting his targets (and did not appear to have any other 'medical' side-effects) then he would support its use. If a universal and medically safe 'teenage contraceptive' that worked through genetic engineering was developed he would be equally happy with that.

Would you, though, be happy working with Mr T? Compared with Marion, Gita and Genevieve he seems to us to be almost a kind of monster! They have their views, but it seems it might be possible to get into a dialogue with them. Hopefully they would be prepared to be self-critical about the value judgements they make, listen to one another's arguments, and possibly even revise them or compromise a little. (Of course, this may not happen. They may hold on to their views dogmatically. You might say that their preparedness to argue for, and be self-critical about their views, is what means we should take them seriously – they are more than simply *views* – and we will return to this issue in Section Three.) But Mr T is certainly a dogmatist. He knows what counts and that is the end of the matter. Further, although he claims to be agnostic about values, he obviously has a value system of his own – a system in which medically defined objectives are given absolute priority and everything else is treated as inconsequential.

Mr T tries to side-step the first two layers of ethical issues discussed at the beginning of this section. He wishes to remain 'outside' of ethical debates about either teenage pregnancy or the legitimacy of public policy and health promotion. He wants to reduce the former to calculations of costs and benefits; and the latter to the measurement of effectiveness. As we discussed in Chapter One, however, this is simply not possible: 'health' and 'health promotion' are contested fields and objective calculation and evidence is therefore never enough. Mr T may believe he can escape our first two layers of ethical issues. But even he cannot escape the ethical issues raised in the third layer – the ethics of professional practice. How is Mr T going to deal with all of the many stakeholders in health promotion? How is he going to take them seriously and treat their views and value judgements with respect? Many of them want him to consider – and to take very seriously, as matters of the utmost importance – things which he regards as outside his remit. Should he humour them? Pretend to take what they say on board but ignore it? Perhaps he should, in the spirit of honesty, just refuse to listen? It seems clear to us that his position is a non-starter. Health promotion ethics surely requires, at the very least, the capacity to seriously engage with the value concerns of the many constituencies of health promotion.

People and statistics – the individual or community in teenage pregnancy

What we have called the technician's perspective has built into it a tendency to reduce the individual to a statistic. Individuals, according to this view, matter to the degree that they contribute to the statistics of harm. But this concern with adding up harms and benefits, of seeing the individual through an 'epidemiological lens', is an important influence on health promotion generally (Hawe, Degeling & Hall 1990). We cannot entirely ignore it. What is wrong with Mr T is that he entirely ignores everything else. It is important to recognise that the technical perspective has some advantages. It requires us to be very clear-sighted about why we are doing things. We need to be able to define and measure why something is a problem, and why something else is a 'solution' to it.

For example, it is by no means clear that Mr T would choose to focus upon teenage pregnancy in any case. If we wish to reduce the risks of low birthweight or other medical complications, we should concentrate on improving the health of *all* pregnant mothers for two reasons. First, there is the general principle, sometimes referred to as the 'prevention paradox' (Rose 1992), that overall benefits are normally best achieved by improving the chances of the whole population at risk, rather than by concentrating efforts on the small minority at high risk. Second, even if we were to concentrate on those at higher risk, then both women at the other end of the child-bearing age range, and more especially women who are experiencing material deprivation, irrespective of age, should be the first priority (Enkin, Keirse & Chalmers, 1989). In other words, 'being a teenager' is not a suitably sensitive indicator of risk for the medical problems we have described above.

A similar argument would apply if our chief concern was to tackle some of the perceived 'social ills' listed above – for example, unmarried motherhood or absent fatherhood. If these were our targets, why focus on teenage pregnancy as opposed to pregnancy outside of marriage? It seems that more is in play than merely technical judgements about harm reduction. A critical voice might say that what is in play is the relative powerlessness of teenagers. Perhaps the moralising 'messages' of social control can be applied more easily to them. A more paternalistic voice might say that it is about the need to protect young people from the 'pains' and responsibilities of pregnancy and give them a chance to build their lives. The fact that teenagers might be more accessible to influence, through educational settings and so on, is simply a fortunate contingency. Both these voices – the critical and the paternalistic – have some plausibility.

Let us accept, for the sake of argument, that there is some sense in having an age of sexual consent, presently 16 for heterosexuals according to law in the United Kingdom. Thus sexual and reproductive freedom under this age is legally forbidden, regardless of any ethical views we might hold. (We *must not* accept sexual activity under this age, which is quite different from the ethical statement that *we ought not* to accept it.) Let us also suppose that women who are in their very early twenties do not have any particular social pressure imposed on them with regard to their sexual and reproductive freedom. (We are not, after all, confronted by newspaper headlines screaming about the social ills created by a wave of pregnant twenty-somethings.) We are then faced with this question: Is there any good reason to treat 16–19 year olds differently from others when it comes to sexual and reproductive freedom? Most people would be very cautious about the way they gave advice and education to a 21 year old woman. If, because of her relatively poor circumstances, she was at a higher risk of having a low birthweight child or a child that grew up in relatively deprived circumstances, most of us would not think to use these facts to try to 'persuade' her from becoming pregnant or having a baby. We might think it was worth her having some information about specific risks but we would not want to try and do any more than that. Why should a 17 year old be treated differently?

There are at least three possible positions here. Which is closest to your own reaction?

(1) *No social pressure should be brought to bear at either age. This is simply moralising. Educational and other service interventions should be designed to allow and support choice about sexuality and pregnancy. In particular the individual woman's choice should not be explicitly set against the contribution she might make to the public health by 'taking the risk' of having a relatively less healthy and happy child.*

(2) *It is perfectly appropriate to bring some pressure to bear in both cases. Educational and other service interventions should be designed to place the responsibility on men and women not to 'take the risk' of having a relatively less healthy and happy child. They might be reminded of the negative impact that 'selfish' decisions can have on the public health or social fabric as well as on the well-being of their children; and benefits and services might be designed to give them disincentives for acting irresponsibly.*

(3) *There are some clear-cut, age-related differences between 17 year olds and 21 year olds which require them to be treated differently. These entitle us to exert more kinds of influence and pressure on the sexual and reproductive freedom of the former than the latter.*

As the local co-ordinator who is trying to tackle teenage pregnancy – or someone involved in this work – you will have some influence on the design and 'tone' of relevant education and services. You will be need to be aware that this is an area permeated with moralising and moral panic. You will need to be able to deal with colleagues who wish to confine themselves to a 'pure' technical perspective. You will have stakeholders like Marion, Gita and Genevieve, and many more, with whom you need to negotiate. Whatever you do, you will be implementing and co-ordinating *some* value judgements and trying to balance conflicts of interests. This is an awesomely difficult challenge. Having read this chapter you might at least test yourself, and everyone with whom you deal, with the following question: Why is teenage pregnancy a problem? The answers to this will suggest very different ways forward. How far, for example, is the agenda related to the well-being of teenagers, or preventive health care, or a vision of a better society? How can you help strike a balance between these and potentially many other agendas, in principle and in practice?

Chapter 5
Do We Know What We're Doing?
Evidence and the Ethics of Lifestyle Change

Introduction

In Chapters Three and Four we have focused on the relationship between health promoters and their 'clients'. Should (we have asked) these relationships be seen broadly as empowering or controlling ones? And we have also looked beyond individual relationships to consider how the work of health promoters might be affected and influenced by broader community concerns. In each case, the challenge for the health promoter is to strike a balance: on the one hand between 'offering help' and 'pressing for change'; on the other between individual and community goals. In this chapter, we bring to centre stage an aspect of debate about health promotion which can dramatically affect the way we assess the ethics of health promotion interventions. Broadly, we want to ask: if there is doubt about whether health promotion actually works, what difference does this make to ethical assessment of our interventions and activities? Or to put in another way: If we are uncertain about the 'evidence' for our work, should we be doing it at all?

The relevance of 'evidence'

In order to get a sense of the importance of these sorts of questions for the process of ethical evaluation, we begin by returning to two earlier examples.

(1) In the introduction to this section, we imagined an NHS hospital trust implementing a no-smoking policy on its premises. This policy will prevent both patients and staff from smoking in almost all parts of the hospital. For example, patients will not be able to smoke in the day rooms of wards or in corridors. If they want to smoke, they will have to go outside the main hospital entrance, possibly suffering the critical gaze of others going in and out. ('If she's in hospital, why on earth is she still smoking?') Nursing and other staff who smoke will not be able to do so in their breaks unless they use a tiny and rather shabby room set aside for the purpose. The room never seems to get cleaned and is at the opposite

end of the hospital to the canteen. ('I'm desperate for a cigarette but I've only got 15 minutes' break.') Clearly, the policy is going to cause inconvenience and possibly distress to a significant minority of those who use or work in the hospital. Let's say the policy was introduced at least partly in order to encourage those who smoke to quit the habit (granted, let us say, that smoking is a health-harming behaviour). Now add to this scenario the following statement: *We don't really know whether smoking policies help people stop smoking.*

(2)   Also in the introduction to this section, we discussed the case of Bob Jones, the heavy drinker admitted to the surgical ward for investigations related to gastric pain. Imagine that the staff nurse discharging him counsels him strongly to significantly reduce his levels of drinking, warning that the risk of not doing so will be increasing levels of serious ill health. Mr Jones is worried by this, but equally worried at the prospect of 'having to do something' about his drinking – his mates at the pub are really his only source of social contact. Let's now add this statement to the scenario: *We don't know whether Mr Jones's current bout of ill-health has anything to do with his drinking; and the debate about what levels of drinking are 'sensible' has been strongly contested over recent years.*

What difference do these additional statements make? At the very least, introducing the idea that there is doubt about whether the interventions 'will work' is likely to make us think again about what we are doing. It may even cause us to want to stop what we are doing, if we are able. To some extent, decisions to modify or stop action will be pragmatic. If we don't know whether what we are doing is working, why should we continue to waste valuable time, energy and, more than likely, financial resources? But this reaction also has an important ethical dimension. Doubt about whether or not health promotion works centrally affects whether we view the field and its activities as ethically acceptable. The prime reason for promoting health is the belief that good or benefit is produced. If we are not confident that our work will produce this benefit, and noting that it will necessarily involve 'costs' of one sort or another, should we be doing it at all?

The nature of the debate on evidence and health promotion

In some areas of life the question of whether what is being done works is relatively simple to answer. When I do my weekly food shopping at the supermarket, or travel to work on the train, or go out to see a film at the cinema, I know whether the service I am using is 'working'. My judgements might be imperfect, and sometimes they will be qualitative and complex, but I will be able to make them relatively simply.

There is much more difficulty in making claims about whether health promotion 'works' or not. Let us review the statements we added to scenarios above:

(1)   We don't really know whether smoking policies help people stop smoking

We do not want directly to address whether this statement is true or not (although at some point it would be crucially important to do so). We want to ask some other questions. What is the person making this statement seeking evidence in relation to? What kind of evidence would satisfy them?

The answer to the first question is quite straightforward. It is asking for information about the effect of smoking policies on smokers' habits. It is asking whether a particular intervention has a particular effect. If we want to dispel doubt, we will have to find out quite a lot. We will want to know, for example, whether smoking policies have been shown to be successful in reducing smoking, how they compare with other health promotion interventions aimed at reducing smoking and so on. This leads to the second question. Presumably the sort of evidence that would satisfy our sceptic (let's assume they are very hard-nosed) would be quite limited. It would have to be evidence that the intervention alone (that is, the implementation of the policy) reduced smoking. Such evidence is likely to be hard to come by for all kinds of reasons, but there is one we want especially to point to here. Smokers, like everyone else, do not live their lives in isolation. They are subject to a range of competing influences, suggestions and pressures. Imagine we are able to discover that 20 members of the hospital staff who previously smoked have given up the habit since the introduction of the smoking policy. How do we know this was directly the result of the policy? Of course we can ask the quitters, but simply by asking them we may alter their perceptions of influences. (And, in any case, we cannot be entirely sure that individuals know precisely what has influenced them.) There is no obvious way of 'controlling' for the effect of this kind of intervention. This problem applies across the whole range of health promotion interventions, simply because these interventions inevitably interact with peoples' social lives and the multiple pressures and influences existing within them.

But it could be that if people give up smoking, they do so because they have been subject to a range of influences including the smoking policy. Other possible influences are levels of tobacco tax, restrictions on cigarette advertising, work by primary health care professionals on individual behaviour change (such as we discussed in Chapter Three) and so on. Indeed, the possibility of multiple influences on health behaviour and how these will be considered and managed by individuals is implicit in models of behaviour change, like the so-called 'Stages of Change' model (Lawrence 1999). Practically, there is some suggestion that the kinds of interventions described above work in a sort of synergy with each other, with the effects of one magnified by the presence of another (Reid *et al.* 1992). If this is so, then decisions about continuing or abandoning the policy should not be taken without trying to consider the 'knock-on' effect of action on other interventions. Understanding these multiple interactions is obviously very difficult and poses a problem for the sceptic. So answering the question about whether the smoking policy 'works' is very hard: both because of our limited capacity to 'control' for the effect of the intervention (people don't live their lives like that); and because it may well be that the intervention is not simply a 'one shot' case of success or failure (health promotion interventions don't work like that).

(2)   We don't know whether Mr Jones's current bout of ill-health has anything to do with his drinking; and the debate about what levels of drinking are 'sensible' has been strongly contested over recent years

Mr Jones was the heavy drinker admitted to hospital with gastritis. The question we need to ask here is: What do we know about the relationship between Mr Jones's present 'unhealthy' state and his drinking habits? Of course, there is good reason to suppose that in drinking several pints of beer each night, Mr Jones is not doing himself any good. The effects of alcohol consumption on general health are well-documented (Knowledge House 1992, Royal College of Physicians 1987). However, it is not easy to argue that the relationship between alcohol consumption and disease onset is a causal one, both in the specific case of Mr Jones and more generally (this more general doubt is implicit in the second part of the statement above).

Let us develop the Mr Jones scenario a bit further. For him, as for anyone, drinking alcohol is only one part of his life – albeit an important part. When he was admitted to the hospital ward, he was asked a number of questions about his 'lifestyle' – diet, smoking and levels of physical exercise, as well as alcohol consumption. The way in which the questions are constructed on the nursing admission form, as well as the way Mr Jones responded to them, meant that the one feature of his health-related lifestyle which emerged prominently was his drinking. Mr Jones was asked if he smoked – he doesn't. When asked about his diet, he told the admitting nurse that it was 'normal' (that is, he wasn't vegetarian or following any other particular diet). This was what was recorded on the admission sheet. In fact, Mr Jones's 'normal' diet consists of a relatively large intake of convenience and 'junk' foods, high in fat. The question on levels of physical activity was: 'Do you take regular exercise?' Mr Jones's answer to the nurse was, 'I walk to and from the station on my way to work.' So the nurse recorded 'Yes'. In fact, Mr Jones's walk to the station is five minutes, never done briskly. For all his working day and for much of weekends, he is sedentary.

A consequence of Mr Jones's high fat, low activity lifestyle is that he is rather (although not considerably) overweight. Weight recording appears on another page of the nursing admission form, which once completed, those giving care may not turn to. What is not asked about at all on this form are perceived levels of stress and psychological tension (at least partly because they are hard to quantify). In fact, Mr Jones is under considerable pressure at the moment, facing the possibility of redundancy and in the middle of marital difficulties.

Why have we gone into such detail about this scenario? It is because a casual glance at Mr Jones's admission sheet would not identify that he had a high fat diet, took hardly any exercise causing physical exertion and was currently leading a pretty stressful life. All it definitely shows in terms of what we might call 'surveillance of negative lifestyle' is that Mr Jones drinks four pints of beer a night, or 56 units of alcohol a week. Consequently, and understandably, the staff nurse chose strongly to counsel him about his drinking. Yet any or all of the other 'risk factors' which have been 'ignored' might equally have contributed to his present ill-health. The point is partly that in Mr Jones's case, the choice to focus on drinking was based on limited evidence and therefore to some extent arbitrary; but it is also that a definitive causal connection between Mr Jones's gastritis and his excessive drinking (or any of the other 'risk factors' mentioned) cannot be established. To suggest that drinking is the cause denies importance to the others. There is a need to be careful about giving any single risk factor a dominant role in explanation. In relation to much disease, causality is difficult to prove (McCormick & Skrabanek 1988).

There is another question to be asked here: how 'risky' is a 'risk factor'; and how is this determined? In asking this question we have in mind a number of background assumptions. First, human beings naturally degenerate – it is the nature of the ageing process, the cycle of life itself. Second, there are certain activities we all have to carry out in order to remain alive – among these are eating and drinking (although admittedly not drinking alcohol). Third, there are some things we are strongly inclined to do because they give us pleasure, or release from an otherwise difficult world. These would include (for large numbers of people) drinking alcohol and smoking. Fourth, some believe there is a connection between some of the things we are inclined to do and morbidity and premature mortality. This belief is a strong basis of much government health promotion policy (Secretary of State for Health 1999). On this basis, it is supposed that the challenge for health promotion is to reduce morbidity and premature mortality through planning and implementing interventions which effectively reduce 'risky' kinds of behaviour, or 'risky' levels of a particular behaviour (McCormick 1994).

But given that either we must engage in some of these behaviours in order to stay alive; or we want to do so in order to make our lives rather more pleasurable or less tedious, we return to the above question. How 'risky' is a 'risk factor'; and how is this determined?

There is dispute about the extent to which alcohol plays a part in the development of disease. Certainly, chronic and continuing abuse of alcohol is likely over time to lead to morbidity and, quite possibly, mortality. The link between alcohol consumption and mortality from cirrhosis (a marker of population alcohol damage) is clear (Knowledge House 1992). Further, reviews (for example, Anderson *et al.* 1988) have examined the results of numerous epidemiological studies which appear to suggest there is evidence of a dose-relationship (that is, the amount drunk) and risk to health. Among other things, excessive alcohol consumption is linked to cirrhosis of the liver, cancers of the oropharynx, larynx and oesophagus, raised blood pressure and stroke.

The picture though, is not quite as simple as this. In thinking about alcohol as a risk factor for stroke, and for coronary heart disease (CHD), the waters start to muddy. Several studies have indicated that drinking some alcohol each day might actually have a protective effect on the heart. Famously, Marmot *et al.* (1981) identified a 'U-shaped curve' for 10-year mortality among civil servants from both cardiovascular and non-cardiovascular causes according to alcohol consumption. This study suggested that risk of mortality decreased somewhat with 'moderate' alcohol consumption, apparently to rise again with 'excessive' drinking. And in a widely publicised study analysing data from the World Health Organisation (WHO), a 40% reduction in the risk of CHD was reported in subjects who drank more than 21 units of alcohol a week (Renaud & De Lorgeril 1992). (A 'unit' of alcohol is a half pint of ordinary strength beer: or a small glass (125 ml) of wine; or a small glass (50 ml) of sherry or port; or a single measure (25 ml) of spirits (Health Education Authority 1993). At the time, 21 'units' was the recommended 'safe' drinking level for men, and 14 for women.)

Some British health promotion opinion has dismissed this ambiguous picture. Indeed, the first national strategy for health for England set tough targets for reducing alcohol consumption, without any reference to the difficulties with the 'evidence' we have indicated (Secretary of State for Health 1992). There seemed, in fact, to be a tendency to ignore these problems. One of the conclusions it might be possible to draw from what has been uncovered is that 'moderate' drinking could have some protective effect from certain cancers and CHD; while 'excessive' consumption is generally damaging to health. So it could reasonably be thought that the health promotion strategists would want to concentrate their efforts on heavy drinkers. Reflect, though, on the following quotation from an officially-sponsored health promotion manual for GPs, produced to support work towards 'The Health of the Nation':

'Which Patients to Target

'In population terms, it is not necessarily the alcohol-dependent and heavy drinkers who are at greatest risk from alcohol – more problems are created by the many moderate drinkers, because there are more of them...' (Knowledge House 1992)

This quotation reflects the well known difference between a focus on 'relative risk' and a focus on 'aggregate benefit' – preventing serious harm to a very few people may not 'do as much good' as preventing moderate harm to many. (Sometimes called the paradox of prevention (Rose 1992)). But in this case the paradoxical position is that evidence of the health benefit to be gained from cutting down on drinking seems to be least convincing in relation to 'moderate drinkers'; yet this is the group which it is suggested should be targeted for health promotion work simply 'because there are more of them . . .'.

Imagine if we were to replace 'alcohol' and 'drinking' in the sentence above with 'food' and 'eating' so that it became:

> 'In population terms, it is not necessarily people addicted to food and those who are obese who are at greatest risk from food – more problems are created by the many moderate eaters, because there are more of them . . .'.

This replacement is not as strange as it might sound. Of course 'moderate drinking' can cause problems (for example, someone could drink two pints, become fuzzy-headed and fall off their bicycle on the way home from the pub); but so can 'moderate eating' (I might eat a modest meal from a local take away and consequently suffer a violent bout of food poisoning). The case for 'risk' in 'moderate eating' is as real as it is in 'moderate drinking'. Indeed, in some respects, the risks we face from food are arguably more extensive than those we face from alcohol – at 'moderate' levels of consumption anyway. We can easily think of 'food scares' such as BSE, but probably find it hard to think of generalised 'scares' to do with the quality and safety of the alcohol many of us drink. We all have to eat in moderation; and many of us derive pleasure from drinking alcohol in moderation. The evidence for dramatically changing habits in relation to one is as convincing (or as unconvincing) as it is for the other. Why, then, should the sentence about 'eating' appear more odd to us than the sentence about 'drinking'?

It is partly, of course, because eating is a necessity; while drinking alcohol (barring cases of addiction, which we are excluding here) is an optional pleasure. But this is only a part of the reason. It seems to us that the concern about alcohol is fundamentally connected to worries about the social effects of widespread and excessive drinking. When we think about 'excessive drinking' nowadays, it is perhaps less likely that it will conjure up images of lone, possibly destitute, alcoholics; and more likely that we will have in our minds pictures of youngsters involved in rowdy and violent weekend nights in the towns of 'Middle England'. 'Teenage drinking' has become almost as potent a symbol of our social ills as 'teenage pregnancy'. On the basis of evidence of the effects of 'moderate' drinking on, say, CHD health, the case for health promotion trying to regulate lifestyle (that is to say, limit drinking) is quite slender (and this is the explicit context in which the advice to GPs above was written). On the basis of wider perceptions, and of values stemming from these – that alcohol can cause social damage which we must limit because we value certain forms of social structures and relationships – then of course the health promotion 'case' for intervening in drinking becomes much stronger and might be expressed something like this:

'Which Patients to Target

'In population terms, it is not necessarily the alcohol-dependent and heavy drinkers who are at greatest risk from alcohol. *Society as a whole is, if we allow moderate drinking to get out of hand. Sometimes, individuals let this happen themselves. The only sensible health promotion strategy, therefore, is to manage moderate drinking so that less people are likely to reach the stage where it might become excessive drinking. We must therefore target all drinkers, no matter how little alcohol they consume . . .'*

On the basis of conflicting epidemiological evidence, certainly in relation to CHD and alcohol, this is all the strategists can say. They must turn their rationale for action into one stemming from particular values, and particular views about the capacity people have to control themselves. In doing so, while the statement becomes much more honest, it also becomes more alarming. ('Why should they try and interfere with me? I enjoy a drink every now and then. I'm quite able to decide when I've had enough.')[2]

Thinking about these examples – smoking policy and sensible drinking – draws out some of the key issues about the nature of evidence in relation to health promotion. We are presented with two broad kinds of problem. First, we may not know (possess sufficient evidence about) the nature of the relationship between health actions and ill-health outcomes (the problem of causation). Second, we may not know (possess sufficient evidence about) whether a particular health promotion action actually works (the problem of intervention).

Is evidence in health promotion different?

There are some who would claim the nature of health promotion 'evidence' makes debate in this area markedly different from such debates in relation to other aspects of health care – 'mainstream' medical practice, for example. To some extent this seems right. After all, part of our purpose in Section One was to

---

[2] The idea that alcohol-related health promotion is used as a method of social regulation – rather than disease prevention – is borne out by recent events. For a sustained period, the upper limits for 'sensible' drinking (14 'units' per week for women and 21 for men) had been established as a result of professional consensus (for example, RCGP, 1986: RCP, 1987). In December 1995, the then Conservative Government announced new guidelines which raised the limits to 21 'units' for women and 28 for men. Yet no new evidence had been uncovered in support of this and the Royal College of Physicians complained at the time that 'by raising the "sensible limits", people are being encouraged to drink more . . .' (Fitzpatrick 2001). The reasons for this government action can only be guessed at, but they appear to have little to do with strategies for preventing disease based on epidemiological evidence.

stake out the distinctiveness of the field of health promotion: the difficulty in specifying the 'ends' and the 'means' of health promotion (and the degree to which they can be contested); its frequently proactive (rather than reactive) nature and so on. This distinctiveness carries through to debates about health promotion evidence. Furthermore, some models of medical science and its evaluation exist which see it as well defined and grounded, and which seem to be dramatically different to the rather fuzzy and disputed picture of health promotion we have built up. For example:

> 'Medical science understands the human body as a complex physical system which becomes dysfunctional when affected by disease ... Its use of the pathogenic as an explanation for health and disease leads to a concern with eliminating those pathogens from the human body or minimising their effects. In order to understand how different curative interventions affect a particular pathogen, evaluative medical research uses experimental designs that test a specific hypothesis and seek to reduce uncertainty about the links between variables...' (Webb 1999).

Nevertheless, it is important to recognise that the picture of objective and scientific certainty about medical practice and its outcomes is to some degree a caricature. While some medical interventions and actions have been evaluated and proven according to the experimental design model – the Randomised Controlled Trial (RCT) – many have not. Even in 'hard' medicine, there are 'hierarchies' of evidence for actions and interventions (Webb 1999) and in some cases little evidence at all. Further, current policy in relation to 'mainstream' medical practice recognises that the complexity of health care structures means that what 'works' in a service in one location will not necessarily work in another (Scally & Donaldson 1998). To see a clear line separating incontestable medical evidence from the highly disputed area of evidence for health promotion is wrong.

The 'Have a Heart at Work' Road Show: the impact of disputes about evidence on the ethics of health promotion

Having thought in a general sense about difficulties with health promotion evidence, we can now return to the question we asked earlier in the chapter: if we are not confident that our work will produce the intended good, should we be doing it at all? This is a question of ethics and we want to consider it against an extended case study.

The study returns us to Otterbury, the town in Southern England where in Chapter Three we examined the work of Vicky Bevan, the practice nurse. Otterbury is home to the headquarters of Ottershire Provident, a life insurance firm with 3000 employees. While the company operates across the UK and abroad, most of these employees work from the Otterbury head office, a large modern building close to the town centre. Much of the work carried out here confines people to their desks. This includes those who work in the company's main call centre, which is sited in the head office.

The insurance industry has a reputation for being highly competitive and in general has undergone waves of mergers, take-overs and de-mutualisations as the market and the way it is regulated changes. Throughout this, Ottershire Provident has remained independent and mutual, although a couple of times recently whispers have gone about in the financial world that it is being sized up by a larger company. The firm has its roots in the nineteenth century, when a number of nonconformist churchmen banded together to make financial provision for their families and friends. Although it is now a big business, the current Chairman and Board of the company try to carry on the ethos of co-operation and mutuality with which it started 150 years before. This attempt forms part of the business's marketing strategy – 'Caring about Insurance and Investment, Caring for You' – but there is also a genuine element of concern for employee welfare. One of the ways in which this is demonstrated is through an occupational health service which has access to the part-time services of a doctor and is headed by a Senior Occupational Health Nurse, Gwen Chapman, who has just taken up the job following the retirement of the previous post holder.

Ottershire, in common with many other parts of England, has a specialist health promotion service, part of the NHS, whose purpose is to support, encourage and co-ordinate health promotion work in the local area. It is particularly concerned to help in the development of activity aimed at promoting health in primary health care, schools and the work place. The health promotion specialist with particular responsibility for the work place is Carol Reilly. She has good connections with some local employers, including the local authority, Otterbury District Council, but not so far with Ottershire Provident. This is partly because Gwen Chapman's predecessor took the view that an occupational health service ought to be largely reactive – about dealing with work place health problems when they arose – rather than engaging in proactive health promotion work. One Wednesday morning, Carol Reilly arrives at work to find, among other things, a letter from Gwen Chapman:

Ottershire Provident ✧ Provident House ✧ PO Box 128 ✧ Otterbury ✧ OB1 1ST

Ottershire Health Promotion Service
Chase House Hospital
Otterbury
OB2 9JD

Dear Sir or Madam

I am writing to you as Senior Occupational Health Nurse at Ottershire Provident. Since I came into the post six months ago, I have been increasingly worried about the lack of attention our company pays to actively promoting the health of the staff. You may know that we employ 3000 people, most at our headquarters here in Otterbury. A large number of these are in very sedentary occupations. I recently conducted a 'mini-health survey' in our offices and from the sample who replied, I was surprised to discover that more than half said they did little or no exercise. Roughly the same number felt that their diet was not as healthy as it could be. About a quarter said they were slightly or moderately worried about their drinking. And about 30% of those who answered said they smoked. It seems to me that we have a heart disease time bomb ticking away among our work force!

I have presented the results of the survey to our senior management team and they have asked me to organise a health promotion programme to address the problem. What I would like to do is to run a 'Have a Heart at Work' Roadshow. I attach the draft of a flier for this and would be grateful for your support. Perhaps some of your health promotion specialists could staff one or two of the road show stands and you may have other ideas about the help you could give.

I hope you will agree this is an important way in which the health of a significant section of the Otterbury work force can be promoted and look forward to hearing from you before long.

Yours faithfully

Gwen Chapman
Senior Occupational Health Nurse

The draft flier is attached to the letter:

'HAVE A HEART AT WORK'

Would you like to feel fitter, be healthier, maybe even live longer?

We are running a special 'Have a Heart at Work' Roadshow in the staff restaurant on Tuesday 24 June from 10 AM to 4 PM. Its aim is to help you to better health.

If you decide to come along, we will weigh you, measure your height and blood pressure and take a finger prick blood sample to check your cholesterol level. Then you will be able to get advice from a number of Roadshow stands which will be staffed by a nurse or a health promotion specialist. They will cover aspects of your life style – eating, drinking, exercise, smoking and so on.

We will organise follow-up sessions after the Roadshow to discuss the results of your cholesterol test and to see how you are getting on with the advice you were given at the 'Have a Heart at Work' Roadshow!

We hope you will want to come. Please reply to this invitation through your line manager so that he or she knows and is able to organise the work of your department or section to cover you.

Carol reads the letter and flier through again, then puts them on her desk. After difficulties with Ottershire Provident in the past, she is pleased to have been approached by the company. But she is worried by what Gwen Chapman has written. It is not so much the practical problems of sorting out help and resources – she is able to do that. Indeed, her manager would encourage the work, given the work place is one of the 'target settings' for the health promotion service. It is more that the work raises important ethical questions for her.

Carol trusts and respects the opinion of her manager, David Gillespie. She decides to go and see him to discuss her worries and arranges to do so later that day:

David: *Hi, Carol, how are you?*
Carol: *Hi, David. Thanks for sparing the time.*
David: *That's OK. Come and sit down. How can I help?*
Carol: *(Sitting in the other comfy chair opposite David's) I've had an approach from Gwen Chapman, the new occupational health person at Ottershire Provident. She wants us to go in and help with some work she's planning.*
David: *Great, that makes a change. So you want some help with it? Maybe you could get Sharma involved. I think she'd be good . . .*
Carol: *Well, yes, but . . . The truth is, David, I'm a bit worried about what Gwen wants to do.*

David: *Worried?*

Carol: *Yes.*

David: (After a pause) *OK. Tell me more.*

Carol: (Passing Gwen's letter and the draft flier for the Roadshow to David) *These are the details. I haven't done anything about it yet.*

David: (After reading the letter and the flier) *So be a bit more specific about what's worrying you.*

Carol: *Alright, here goes. Basically, I think there are problems with both why Gwen's planning to do this; and with what she's planning to do.*

David: *You mean with the motivations of the company?*

Carol: *No, not really, although I suppose you could start to get worried about work place health surveillance and power structures and all that sort of stuff. But you know me, David – I'm enough of a pragmatist to accept that all that might be going on but at the end of the day there's still a good opportunity actually to promote health. The problem here is that I'm not convinced there is that opportunity.*

David: *I never thought I'd hear you call yourself a pragmatist!*

Carol: (Laughing) *Times change. But there's limits to my pragmatism.*

David: *OK. But why are there limits here? Why shouldn't this kind of thing improve health? Simple checks on weight and cholesterol and stuff. Advice on diet and exercise and smoking and drinking. It's your good basic health promotion.*

Carol: *I know. And that's why I'm reluctant to criticise it. Plus this is a place we've wanted to work with for a long time. But if you really think about what Gwen's planning to do, it doesn't quite hold up. Can I have the stuff she sent me back for a minute?*

David: (Passing the letter and the flier back to Carol) *Sure.*

Carol: *Thanks. Now think about this.* (Reading and paraphrasing from the flier) *'Would you like to feel fitter, be healthier, maybe even live longer?... Blah blah... The Roadshow's aim is to help you to better health... Blah blah... If you come, we will ... check your cholesterol level and give you advice on ... eating, drinking, exercise and smoking...'. It all sounds quite simple. In essence, what the flier's saying is let us do some elementary tests, give you some advice and you can avoid CHD. Or at least minimise the risks. It's a perfect justification. If we do this work, benefit will result – not so many people will suffer from heart disease.*

David: *Aha. Your 'famous principles'. I was starting to wonder when they would appear.*

Carol: (Slightly defensive) *There's nothing wrong with principles. If you do health promotion, I mean, if you do it because you believe it's a good thing for there to be 'more health' for more people, then why shouldn't you try and think about whether what you're doing is likely to produce benefit?*

David: (Slightly chastised) *I'm sorry. You're right. Carry on.*

Carol: *OK. The implication of this flier is 'We find out this ... you do that ... this will happen.' It suggests that there's a causal connection between all these risk factors and someone getting CHD.*

David: *But in the case of smoking, that's pretty much so, isn't it? I mean, there's been* *studies like Framingham and the British Regional Heart Study[3] showing smoking's associated with a two- to three-fold increase in CHD risk, compared with not smoking. And for stroke, the risk is at least doubled. And we haven't even started to talk about cancer . . .*

Carol: *I agree. In fact, smoking is the 'risk factor' I probably have the least difficulty with here. It's quite right to say to people, stop smoking or don't start and your risks of lung cancer will be radically reduced. I'd be inclined to say the same thing in relation to CHD, too. But smoking isn't straightforwardly and distinctively causal of heart disease in the way epidemiology shows it to be of lung cancer. The evidence is more conflicting. For example, the North Karelia project in Finland was inconclusive about smoking as a risk marker for CHD. And there have been suggestions that what counts is the combination within a population of high serum cholesterol levels with high smoking prevalence. Countries like Japan, where smoking prevalence is high and serum cholesterol is low, have traditionally had less of a problem with CHD.*

David: *OK. But some of that ambiguity relates to difficulties with the studies them-selves. I mean, long follow-ups are needed to show the full results. Some of what you're talking about may be based on follow-ups that are too short. There's also the problem – even with very well resourced studies and trials – of being able to isolate the impact of interventions on the study group and of being able to stop the control group being exposed to things that would help them reduce their CHD risk anyway – even if the researchers wanted to do that. And I guess you need to remember that it's limiting to talk about an intervention – something around smoking advice, say – just having an effect on heart disease mortality. Surely there's going to be general health benefits.*

Carol: *Oh yes, like I said, smoking's probably the thing I take least issue with here. Although if I was being awkward I would probably argue that the way this 'Have a Heart Roadshow' is being framed gives the strong impression that stopping smoking means in every case, all the time, reducing the risk of CHD.*

David: *But then it's down to the people giving advice to make the thing less black and white and more shades of grey, isn't it?*

Carol: *Yes. Except if you want my opinion, health promotion (at least 'official' health promotion) doesn't have much of a reputation for presenting things in shades of grey. And things become more grey if you think about some of the other risk factors Gwen Chapman's planning to work on.*

David: *You're going to talk about alcohol now, aren't you?*

Carol: *No it's alright, David, I'll give that a miss. You know what I'd say on the basis of our planning meetings for the last Drinkwise campaign.*

David: *(Smiling) Those meetings are etched on my memory, Carol.*

Carol: *(Smiling too) I thought they might be. No, let me just talk about one other thing. Cholesterol and diet. Because I think here things become much more problematic,*

---

[3] Carol's and David's discussion is detailed, but they don't give each other references! To avoid interrupting their dialogue, we give details of the studies, reviews and discussions they refer to at the end of this chapter.

partly because of the lack of convincing evidence about the benefit of change in terms of reducing CHD risk; but also because what Gwen's proposing might actually breach one of my other 'famous principles'.

David: *Go on.*

Carol: *Medical people have spent loads of time since the 1960s trying to scientifically verify the link between diet and CHD risk. I mean, beyond recognition of a plausible thesis of association. You've got a fairly clear aetiological picture – fatty plaques on the lining of coronary arteries form blood clots which in turn cause heart attacks. And the factor linking dietary fat to fatty plaque formation appears to be blood cholesterol levels. So it makes sense to suppose that if you alter intake of dietary fat, you lower levels of blood cholesterol. But the evidence for this is still conflicting. For example, MR FIT . . .*

David: *You mean the Multiple Risk Factor Intervention Trial?*

Carol: *Yes. MR FIT failed to establish any definitive link between risk factor reduction (including dietary change) and heart disease mortality. Another major trial on CHD prevention in the early 1990s actually revealed an increase in mortality among those who'd received a medical intervention, which included help with lowering cholesterol.*

David: *OK, so you could argue that the picture of benefit is ambiguous. There's two things I would argue in return. First, you're talking about individual risk factors in isolation – picking off smoking, or alcohol, or diet. Surely if we work on reducing risk across the range of factors, we will achieve benefit? And second, I go back to something I said earlier. We may find it hard to come up with causal proof that doing x, y or z will reduce your chances of mortality from CHD, but I know very well that if I ate better, cut down on my drinking on occasions and took more exercise, I'd feel better. My sense of well-being would be improved.*

Carol: *(Laughing) And so would mine! Seriously, though, I think both the points you make are connected. Addressing CHD 'risk factors' together may well improve someone's sense of well-being. But that's a very different claim from one that's about suggesting their risk of CHD is definitively diminished (and the implication within this that the connection between risk factor and disease onset is causal). Plus the presentation of what you might call multiple risk factors demands that you try and convey a more complex picture altogether. If someone doesn't smoke but has a poor diet while taking a reasonable amount of exercise, you have to start talking about 'relative risk', of being much less categorical than you might feel you can be if you concentrated on just one thing (even though being categorical might not be at all warranted). You also have to start talking about much more nebulous concepts – like the 'well-being' you mentioned. All this requires time and a respect for autonomy . . .*

David: *Another principle!*

Carol: *Yes. Which might or might not be present in a health promotion intervention. Time will tell on that one, but the signs may not be good. Gwen might be being driven by targets set by her company's board. I mean, they may be more interested in cutting down levels of smoking, say, than in discovering how many of their staff feel their 'well-being' has improved. They're more likely to 'go for' the quick fix of a high profile Roadshow, where people are subjected to brief advice, than a more comprehensive* *programme of different sorts of interventions, all aiming to support and empower employees, and respect their autonomy – even though this kind of programme may be more effective in some respects.*

David: *Well, like you said, we need to wait and see, as well as offer some guidance to Gwen, perhaps. Was it respect for autonomy you meant when you talked before about cholesterol testing and dietary advice breaching another of your ethical principles?*

Carol: *It wasn't actually, although it could have been. In fact, I was thinking of the principle of non-maleficence, of doing no harm.*

David: *What do you mean?*

Carol: *OK, you could argue that cholesterol testing – at least as its planned here by Gwen – is a form of screening. That's when screening is thought of as a method applied to a population of asymptomatic individuals, with nothing to suggest they are at higher risk of the condition or disease being screened for than the rest of the population, with the purpose of selecting for further investigation or treatment. Mant and Fowler suggested that before you embark on screening, you need to ask yourself a number of questions to justify your practice, including: Can you offer effective treatment for patients positive on testing? How many positive tests will prove to be false alarms (and is this acceptable)? How many patients will you need to follow up over the next five years (and can you sustain this work load)? Now there's quite a few issues here for what Gwen's planning. First, 'effective treatment'. If we find out that someone's got a raised cholesterol level, we may try and get them to change their diet. For at least some people, this is actually going to be very difficult and they're going to need support. Is it there? Simple fat-reducing diets of the 'enjoy healthy eating' sort are relatively easy to handle, but they produce very marginal reductions in cholesterol levels. More drastic diets with a greater likelihood of achieving target reductions are grim. And in any case, like I said before, the evidence that reducing dietary fat lowers cholesterol is still conflicting. Second, what do we mean by 'positive tests' and 'false alarms' here? Someone might be discovered to have raised cholesterol, but raised by how much? And at what raised levels are we confident that someone presently asymptomatic in all other respects is heading for CHD? Think again of MR FIT and other trials where interventions appear to have produced little benefit, at least in terms of mortality. Yet now we've got people walking around, worried about their cholesterol levels. We've caused harm. And third, the possibility of harm might be exacerbated if you think about Mant and Fowler's question on follow-up and work load sustainability. You've got about 3000 people working at Ottershire Provident. Assume 10% come to the Roadshow. Assume 10% of those attending are discovered to have levels of cholesterol raised sufficiently to warrant professional help from a dietician. 30 people. It doesn't sound like very much, but I know that Jenny Hudson and the dietetic service are really stretched at the moment – especially with Laura Cole being away on maternity leave. Are they going to be able to cope with even just 30 extra referrals? If there are doubts about the 'effectiveness' of the 'treatment' we're able to offer; if we're not really sure about what we mean by 'positive tests' and 'false alarms'; if we're not sure we can support follow-up for even small numbers through access to specialist services; should we be doing this screening*

at all? We'll be raising anxieties among people we identify as 'at risk' without necessarily being able to do much for them in terms of diminishing risk. We'll be causing
harm.

David: *OK. So what you're saying is that this 'Have a Heart at Work' Roadshow is flawed
in terms of what you might broadly call the evidence supporting it. The relationship
between the things it's looking at (the 'risk factors') and eventual CHD is unclear. And
you don't know whether the kinds of things you're actually going to be doing there – say,
cholesterol testing and consequent dietary advice – will actually have any effect.*

Carol: *That's it.*

David: *I think what we need to do is approach Gwen Chapman very gently with some
possible alternatives . . .*

Conclusion

Of course, as David Gillespie has suggested, there are alternatives. In some
respects, our presentation of the case against the 'Have a Heart at Work'
Roadshow rests on our own selection of 'the evidence': both about the
relationship between CHD risk factors and the disease itself; and about the
effectiveness of interventions, such as cholesterol testing. We have deliberately
emphasised evidence casting doubt on the relationship between risk factors and
disease. But the fact that we have been able to do so suggests that simple messages
such as 'drink sensibly and you won't get CHD' are evidentially problematic.

Perhaps more importantly, we have tended to play down alternative ways in
which the evidence available might be interpreted. In this case study, we have
deliberately amplified the importance of understanding the available evidence in
relation to CHD. As David started to suggest, it might be more helpful to assess it
in terms of more general health benefits. (Although many of the studies Carol and
David were discussing had the explicit aim of providing evidence for heart disease
causation and prevention.) But if we framed our advice on smoking, eating,
drinking and so on in terms of a desire more generally to improve health and well-
being – if, in other words, we widened our conceptions of *how* we were trying to
be effective – we might be less likely to get caught in an ethical trap. This is the
trap of trying to justify our work in terms of its benefit whilst having both a very
rigorous and a narrow conception of 'benefit'.

Of course, having wider conceptions of 'benefit' (and equally of 'harm') brings
its own ethical difficulties. We may be accused on the one hand of being simply
too broad and of not adhering to specific managerial imperatives relating to
disease prevention; or on the other of making assumptions about how the individual clients or communities we serve actually understand, for example, their
'well-being'. Furthermore a concern with wider benefits contains just as much (if
not more) complexity and uncertainty about the nature and quality of evidence
available to underpin our practice. Here – as elsewhere – there is no escape from

ethical difficulties. All we can do is openly acknowledge them, address them to the best of our ability, and be as clear and open as possible about our thinking in the process.

Here are the references which supported the discussion between Carol and David:

Dunnigan, M. (1993) The problem with cholesterol. *British Medical Journal*, **306**, 1355–6.

Gunning-Schepers, L.J., Barendregt, J.J., Van Der Maas, P.J. (1989) Population interventions reassessed. *The Lancet*, 479–81.

Mant, D. & Fowler, G. (1990) Mass screening: theory and ethics. *British Medical Journal*, **300**, 916–18.

Marteau, T. (1990) Reducing the psychological costs. *British Medical Journal*, **301**, 26–8.

Multiple Risk Factor Intervention Trial Group (1982) Multiple risk factor intervention trial. Risk factor changes and mortality results. *Journal of the American Medical Association*, **248**, 1465–77.

NHS Centre for Reviews and Dissemination (1998) Cholesterol and Coronary Heart Disease: Screening and Treatment. *Effective Health Care Bulletin*, **4** (1).

Ramsay, L.E., Yeo, W.W., Jackson, P.R. (1994) Effective diets are unpalatable. *British Medical Journal*, **308**, 1039.

Salonen, J.T., Puska, P., Mustaniemi, H. (1979) Changes in coronary risk factors during a comprehensive five-year community programme to control cardiovascular diseases (The North Karelia Project). *British Medical Journal*. 1178–83.

Shaper, A.G., Pocock, S.J., Walker, M. *et al.* (1981) British Regional Heart Study: cardiovascular risk factors in middle-aged men in 24 towns. *British Medical Journal*, **283**, 179–86.

Thom, T.J., Epstein, F.H., Feldman, J.J., Leaverton, P.E. (1985) Trends in total mortality and mortality from heart disease in 26 countries from 1950 to 1978. *International Journal of Epidemiology*, **14**, 510–20.

Tones, K. & Tilford, S. (1994) *Health Education: Effectiveness and Efficiency (2nd Edition)*. Chapman and Hall, London.

Chapter 6
Who Decides What To Do?
A Food Policy Case

Introduction

In the previous three chapters, we have concentrated upon three key ethical concerns in health promotion decision-making. We have been seeking to explore the tensions between controlling and enabling tendencies: the dilemmas that emerge in attempting to think about both individuals and communities at the same time; and problems related to decision-making in conditions of uncertainty. In the background of all these discussions lies a further concern – one we signalled in Chapters 1 and 2 – which needs to be brought more into the open. Who makes, and who ought to be making, health promotion decisions?

Our discussions so far have been organised around expressions such as 'dilemmas', 'judgements', 'decisions', 'balancing acts' and so on. All of these terms rely upon the idea of agency, of particular agents doing the deciding and acting. They presuppose that we have in mind certain people or organisations who are, so to speak, 'charged' with responsibility for ethical health promotion. Because the main focus of this book is on the professional responsibilities of health promoters (whether health promotion specialists or other health professionals) we have tended to equate agency for health promotion with health promoters. We have – either explicitly or by implication – suggested it is these people who possess the lion's share of both the agency and the responsibility. This emphasis is quite useful in some respects – it underlines the personal and professional responsibilities of those who think of themselves as 'doing health promotion'. By now, however, it should also be clear that it obscures three fundamental matters.

First, all kinds of agencies, including the government and public, private and voluntary organisations have a role in health promotion. Individual citizens have a role too. All of these, arguably, have some share of the responsibility for it. Second, the agency of health promoters is seriously circumscribed. They have to work within frameworks which are only partly within their control. Third, health promoters will typically want to make their decisions in conjunction with the clients or communities they are serving or addressing. Indeed, sharing responsibility for decision-making can be seen as a professional obligation; it is not just something that they want to do, but something that they ought to do.

In discussions about the ethics of health promotion, the question, 'Who decides?' raises a host of overlapping issues. In this chapter we want to focus on some of these issues. In the first two sections of the chapter, we try to map the issues in a conceptual sense. Following this, in the main body of the chapter, we explore them further and in more detail by considering how they show themselves in an example. Our example relates to food policy. Finally we will try to draw these two discussions – conceptual and policy-related – together and discuss their implications for health promotion ethics.

Power, autonomy and responsibility

We all know from first-hand experience that there are connections between power, autonomy and responsibility. In situations where we are relatively powerless our autonomy is limited; and where our autonomy is limited then, we judge, so must be our responsibility for what happens. We can see in reflecting on these connections that they are of conceptual as well as practical importance. Ideas of power, autonomy and responsibility are closely related to each other. In this section we want to review these conceptual relationships and begin mapping out their importance for health promoters.

All decisions are made within systems of power relations. This is a pervasive fact of life. Generally speaking, parents are more powerful than children; employers more powerful than employees; governors more powerful than the governed. In each case the former are likely to have 'more of a say' in decisions than the latter. We say 'generally speaking' because power is situational. Power relations are complex. They shift from context to context, and from agenda to agenda (Fielding 1996). There is no completely stable and definitive hierarchy of power. Nonetheless, in every situation hierarchies exist and many of these hierarchies are relatively stable.

One way of understanding power relations is in terms of the control of individuals (Handy 1985). The word 'control' is in some respects a little crude – it suggests, perhaps, the deliberate and far reaching oppression of individuals – but it captures a core idea. Namely, that in a situation where an individual has power exercised over them, the upshot of such exercise is that their autonomy is compromised to at least some degree. This is the conceptual connection between power and autonomy, and it is worth elaborating a little. For the purposes of this discussion, let us say that an individual is autonomous to the extent that he or she is able to make and enact his or her own choices in his or her life (this is a shorthand summary of many definitions of autonomy). Given this, it seems there are two main types of constraint on autonomy; what might be called internal and external constraints. Internal constraints are those which refer to a lack of capacity to make or enact choices – perhaps because the individual is still an infant, or because they are mentally ill, or dependent on substances. We will not be saying anything about these internal kinds of constraints here. External constraints are those which refer to social and environmental conditions limiting people's ability to make and enact their own choices in lives (and may, of course, play a causal role in the production of at least some kinds of internal constraints).

Sometimes we are not 'allowed' to make certain choices, to express them, or to carry them out. The society in which we live and the people around us can impose various kinds of constraints on our autonomy. Most of these do not involve the crude use of physical force but more subtle mechanisms of rules, norms, rewards and sanctions – even perhaps merely the approval or disapproval of 'significant others' in our lives. These systems of power are not only more or less subtle; they are also more or less overt. Sometimes they are obvious; but sometimes they remain hidden and we may have to be analytical and reflective to bring them to mind. An example of an obvious constraint is when our boss simply tells us what to do without any kind of discussion or negotiation. An example of a hidden constraint might be in discovering that some different priorities have been 'smuggled into' an innocuous looking new policy document. (William Connolly sets out a sophisticated analysis of the various overt and covert faces of power in his *The Terms of Political Discourse* (1993).)

This last example takes us to the heart of the concerns of this chapter. Health promoters are positioned in the middle of chains of power, with policy makers and managers on one side; and the public on the other. They are not only subject to systems of power; they also transmit power and exercise it over others (granted, they are often, through empowerment approaches, attempting to reduce these power imbalances). So in order to see 'Who decides?' we have to consider all the agencies in the chains of influence and power. What is more, if we ask 'Who ought to decide?' we also have to consider the power relations between these agencies. This is because it is misleading to ask 'Who ought?' unless we are able to ask 'Who can?' as well. It is, after all, more than a little odd to say, 'I know Fred is not in a position to do x – but he ought to do x'. (This idea is sometimes summarised in the phrase, 'Ought implies can'.) There is a wide acceptance of the view that health promoters should be cautious before they hold individuals responsible for their unhealthy lifestyle choices – precisely because they may not actually be autonomous choices (Tones & Tilford 1994). For the same reasons, we should be cautious about holding individual health promoters responsible for health promotion practice. Such practice emerges from a compound of interactions between national and local policies, vested interests, managerial and professional cultures, settings and client values. It is not a pure product of the autonomous choices of individual health promoters.

Having made this acknowledgement, we also need to recognise a contrary danger. We cannot – as individual citizens or as professionals – blindly take refuge behind the fact that social processes are complex, and that practices are a result of overlapping and criss-crossing chains of influence. We cannot say, 'I don't know what caused this and therefore I'm not responsible for it!' If a bank robber cites the complexity of social life and social influences as the reason for his crime, or a seriously negligent doctor refers to the same factors as the explanation for his failures, we would have limited patience at best with their explanations. As well as recognising complexity, we also have to recognise some fairly clear lines of responsibility. The ethical shortcomings of, say, the bank robber and the doctor, may be partly a product of their environment. We will usually wish to examine these environmental influences carefully before we come to judgement, and will take them into account when constructing penalties. However, they do not explain the responsibility away. To the extent that individuals are in fact autonomous, we expect them to bear some of the responsibility at least for the foreseeable consequences of their actions. So the conceptual connection between autonomy and responsibility becomes clear. Diminished autonomy entails diminished responsibility, but the reverse also holds true – we cannot claim autonomy and at the same time deny responsibility.

Before ending this section, it is necessary to comment on a problem many health promoters appear to have with the idea of responsibility. They may be quite willing to accept responsibility for their own actions but for very good reasons they are wary of holding clients responsible for shortcomings such people may be perceived as having. Many health promoters do not want to indulge in 'blaming the victim' – this is often a crucial principle within their work (Society of Health Education and Health Promotion Specialists 1997b). At the same time, however, they often want to share responsibility for choices with their clients; to empower them to make choices and to contribute to policy making. On the one hand they wish to 'give' responsibility to others; but on the other they do not wish to 'hold' these others responsible, in the sense of blaming them.

There are some apparent contradictions here which need to be analysed. With all welfare professionals inherent tensions exist between attitudes which arguably 'infantilise' people by treating them as if they are not responsible for their lives; and attitudes which treat them as equal partners with the implication that they might also take some share of the responsibility for what gets done. Yet further analysis suggests there need be no direct contradiction here. We have already discussed a central reason why health professionals should reserve blame for as long as possible. It is simply too difficult to map all of the influences which shape people's lives and actions. Health professionals are there to support – not to judge – and this involves giving people the benefit of the doubt. Part of such support is to help build autonomy and to be ready to respect apparently autonomous choice.

Informed choice in health promotion

The issue we will explore most in this chapter is that of the sharing of power and responsibility for decision-making between health promoters and their clients. In the case of one-to-one encounters between health professionals and their clients, certain norms are fairly widely understood – even if they are not always followed. We would expect the outcome of a doctor-patient or nurse-patient interaction to reflect the values and choices of both parties. The health professional might suggest certain courses of action (particular treatments or lifestyle adjustments say) but we would expect that the client is given a proper opportunity to discuss, consider and agree to whatever is proposed. The language and practices of 'informed consent' or 'informed choice' have grown up to embody these expectations. Patients – and here we are assuming that they are relatively autonomous – require information they can understand and the opportunity to make choices (without any kind of coercion or pressure) about what they will do or about what might be done to them (Gorovitz 1985). In practice, it may not always be easy to see whether these conditions have been properly fulfilled but the standards are relatively clear. Furthermore, this is a necessary minimum for health professional practice. Anyone who falls below these standards will be judged to have been acting unethically. (See, for example, statements related to consent in the United Kingdom Central Council for Nursing's (UKCC) 'Guidelines for Professional Practice' (UKCC 1996).) There are many extra things – above and beyond this minimum – which health professionals who are client-centred will want to do. They will want to listen to the concerns and preferences of the client. They will also want to encourage the client to offer their own solutions. And they will want to give them the chance fully to explore and debate the alternatives in a constructive meeting of minds. These are all ethical ideals many health professionals will subscribe to and they will, in this regard, be better and more admirable professionals for it. To repeat, however – informed choice is not an ideal in health care. It is an ethical requirement.

Can we apply the principles behind informed choice to all aspects of health promotion? Shouldn't we require that client groups (where competent) are fully informed about proposed courses of health promotion action and have a full and free opportunity to agree to them before they are implemented? It is tempting simply to say 'yes', but a closer look at the issues reveals three major factors making it difficult to give an affirmative answer to this latter question. We will set out these difficulties in the remainder of this section in order to complete the background to our case study on food policy.

We do not want to deny that the broad principles behind informed choice can and should be applied to health promotion work. However, there are both theoretical and practical problems in realising these principles when the focus shifts from individuals to populations. It is important that health promoters are ready to share information with their clients. This is a core element of their work. (See, for example, UKCC (1992), Society of Health Education and Health Promotion Specialists (1997b).) In general they should be prepared to make the knowledge base on which they make decisions, and the rationale for those decisions, transparent. For example, if the authorities in a particular area decide they are going to fluoridate the water supply, we would expect them to be ready not only to publicise the decision, but also to explain and justify it to the population of that area. Indeed, we imagine that the population concerned would expect to be consulted before the decision was made. All of these things are highly important ethical expectations that we are right to have of health promoters. However, as this example suggests, they fall short of the model of informed choice we described earlier.

The first problem with applying informed choice to population health promotion is the difficulty of delimiting and defining interventions. Fluoridation is a fairly clear-cut and well defined intervention. (And many other interventions – such as breast cancer screening or Measles, Mumps and Rubella (MMR) vaccination – would also fall into the category of fairly-well defined interventions.) They are deliberate and focused biomedical or environmental measures, introduced to protect or promote population health. But as we have emphasised in different parts of this book, there is an almost endless list of other policies and practices which have some health promotion implications – and which are much less well defined. For example, many transport or environmental policy decisions will have a health-related element to them. Should each and every decision made by national or local governments which have a potential health promotion function be subject to a process of informed choice? This represents not only the difficulty of indefinitely multiplying consultation exercises, it also represents the difficulty of deciding on who consults with whom. Again, as we stressed in Chapter 2, it is often not clear precisely which agents are responsible for 'interventions' and who is affected by them. Increasingly, governments stress the importance of public-private partnerships, inter-agency working and 'joined up solutions'. The practical outcome of this emphasis on the part of government is that clear-cut parties who would be able to forge the 'contract' of informed choice may well not exist.

The second, and more fundamental problem facing informed choice in population health promotion, is the problem of minority belief and preference. Even in those cases where both the intervention and the two parties (agency and population) are well-defined, there is the question of what happens when there is a disagreement within the population concerned. Suppose the authority involved wants to give its population informed choice about fluoridation. And suppose it goes to a lot of expense and trouble to inform the public about the arguments for and against fluoridation, and to respond to all requests for further research and data. Following a period of discussion and debate it organises a poll – 90% vote in favour of fluoridation and 10% vote against it. What should it do? Should it go ahead on the basis that large numbers of the population have given their 'informed consent' to the intervention? Or should it keep things as they are because a substantial proportion of people has refused 'informed consent' to the change? The poll does not settle the matter for the authority – the consultation may be a useful exercise and the views of the public need to be 'taken into account' but it still has to make the decision.

This example shows that the analogy with informed consent is actually rather misleading in this health promotion context. We are not just talking of individuals making a choice about what should happen to them, but of individuals making a choice about a policy issue which will affect many other people. This is a very different matter. It is not obvious that in the normal course of events, person A should have a say about what happens to person B unless person A is authorised to do so in some way. (There may, of course, be circumstances where such authorisation is allowed and has been given: for example, person A is a judge and person B a defendant; or person A is person B's elected representative.) It is possible, perhaps, to advance the idea that 'democracy' allows people to have a say in one another's lives and that for this reason alone person B may be subject to person A's views, where person A is in the majority. However, although this may be true in some instances, most democratic systems only allow for exercises of direct democracy in limited and occasional circumstances. This is the case for the very reasons we have been rehearsing here – democratic systems have to be designed to protect the interests of minorities.

The third difficulty facing the extension of informed choice to population health promotion is the overwhelming practical challenge of establishing the necessary conditions for good quality communication and choice in public decision making. In order to secure informed choice in clinical encounters, we need to know the patient understands the options and is freely expressing their views and preferences. The communication conditions have to be good in order for the health professional to be satisfied about these things. Similarly, there must be proper freedom of choice and expression available to the patient. Putting these conditions in place is not easy, even in the case of individual patient-professional relationships. To establish the social equivalents of these conditions for an exercise in *population* informed choice would be exceptionally taxing. If we return to the fluoride example we can illustrate this difficulty a little. How could the authority concerned satisfy itself that the full population was properly informed about the options? Equally, how could it satisfy itself that it was fully informed about the freely expressed views of the population? Even assuming that we are dealing only with adults of voting age (and of course this is an assumption some would want to question), there is likely to be a very heterogeneous range of people within the population. People will be of different ages, genders and ethnicities. They will have different interests, different levels of access to media, different learning styles and so on. Some of them will be highly literate about science; others will be virtually 'science phobic'. Some will have plenty of time available to consider the issue; others will have no time at all. Many of them may not have English as a first language and will rely on translations or interpreters if they are to properly participate in the public discussion. None of these variations causes a problem of principle – that is to say, they ought not forestall the idea of communication and consultation. However, when they are combined, they do present enormous practical problems for achieving the 'informed' element of informed choice. The 'choice' element causes equivalent problems. The fact that someone may have cast a vote in a certain direction is an indication of a choice but it would not necessarily be considered a sufficient indication of independent voluntary choice. Normally we would like to be able to check that this expression of a preference was based on a proper understanding of what the particular vote meant, and that no undue pressure had been brought on the voters. (Both of these factors have played a part in election controversies. Historically there have been many scandals about votes being 'bought' by vested interests. And one of the concerns about the Florida count in the United States' presidential election of 2000 was simply that voters in some counties had been 'thwarted' by the design of the ballot paper.) To check that these conditions of 'voluntariness' and 'under-standing' have been met for a whole population is likely to be a daunting task and would require, at the very least, a number of in depth 'spot checks'.

These three difficulties, and especially the second one, mean we should be wary about extending the language of informed choice to population health promotion. It is not only practically difficult to implement; it is also in some ways conceptually misleading. Nonetheless the values of sharing information, of supporting understanding, of providing and protecting opportunities for public participation remain of central ethical importance.

Food quality and choice – a case study in food policy

February 18th

Fiona Haddon is a Senior Nurse Manager at St. Alfred's Hospital NHS Trust in Billingham, Hertfordshire. She is currently working on secondment as a Practice Development Nurse and heading up the Practice Development Team, partly to cover a colleague's maternity leave and partly to update her own skills and knowledge. One aspect of her job is to troubleshoot on the wards – to set up mechanisms to respond to, and support the needs of her colleagues. The job is extremely complex. She has more demands to meet than she has available time; for this reason alone, she is a little wary about having agreed to chair a Hospital working group on 'Food Quality and Choice'. While Fiona sees this is an important subject, she is not convinced it is a good use of her time to get involved in another 'talking shop'. The first meeting of the working group is tomorrow. In an effort to save time, she has invited members of the group to let her have any thoughts on what they understand the issues to be in advance of the meeting. She has had four messages from various people and decides to take them home that evening to read them and help collect her thoughts. Here are extracts from the four messages:

From Joanne, the catering manager – *The fact that the Trust's senior management team has put this firmly on the agenda is a really positive development. As you know there are a number of moves both nationally and regionally pushing us to improve the quality and choice of food. I know we use good quality ingredients and I am sure we can make some improvements to the quality of meals. We have already developed a menu card system. This has settled into use now and might easily be extended. It not only provides choice but also gives us a good idea of what is popular and some kind of evaluation when things remain popular over time. Obviously, we would need a substantial injection of extra resources if we are being realistic about extending the system – we will have to adapt our ordering, storage and distribution systems and we will also need to increase the numbers of staff on each shift. The bottom line is that we cannot make improvements without some increase in expenditure. Also, menus must be realistic cost wise. Don't forget that we only have about £2 per head a day to spend! If we plan this carefully and are able to find pump-priming money to plan and introduce the system changes, then the ongoing increases might be relatively small (perhaps only a 5% increase). But the senior management team need to know now that this means money. Otherwise there is no point talking about it.*

From Sudi, a nutritionist – *I don't think that increasing choice, if it's done carefully, will necessarily cause any problems provided we are offering from a range of well balanced meals. The fundamental things are food safety and nutritional quality. We have good working relationships with the catering department and I'm sure we could be involved where appropriate. After all, many patients tend only to eat what they want to eat in any case. Of course there are always some for whom managing their food intake is an important aspect of their treatment and we may have to restrict their choice of food to some extent. But this is the exception rather than the rule. Generally, though, I feel we should pay attention to our health promotion function in constructing food choices. We are in a position to 'model' a healthy diet for our population, and we should take this seriously – but of course part of doing this is to show that a good diet needn't be boring or puritanical.*

From Danny, a research nurse – *As you know I am undertaking a small exploratory study of patients' perceptions and wants concerning food. It will be a few weeks before I've properly analysed my data but I can give you some quick feedback if it helps. Bear in mind that this is only based on 20 interviews and there is no way they can be representative of all patients. However I passionately believe that we should be starting from the patients' perspective here. There are limits to how far they can make other decisions – but surely they can make decisions about the hospital's food policy.*

So far I think three main themes seem to be emerging:

First, there are those who have come up with 'wish lists' of food choice. For example people have suggested that there should be a ready supply of pizzas or filled baguettes as well as the traditional meals. Many people have mentioned more curry availability – the nation's favourite dish. When people get going on these lists there is a general sense that there are quite a lot of food options readily available on the high street but much less available in the hospital.

Second, there are those for whom food is a self-conscious part of their identity and for whom food choice is a moral and political question. This includes vegetarians and vegans, and those with religion-related dietary requirements. These individuals all understandably want to ensure that the Trust at least caters for their specific needs and ideally offers them more choice, too. One vegetarian expressed the view that he was 'a second class citizen' as far as the hospital was concerned. I also spoke to a couple of people who expressed more overtly political views – one arguing that the hospital should not offer meat as an option because it was colluding in the suffering and murder of animals; and one saying that the hospital should take a stand against genetically modified food.

Third, and following on from this, many people said they did not want to eat certain things – GM food and beef in particular. They wanted, so to speak, the choice not to eat those things.
I hope this is food for thought!

From Kevin, a senior administrator – *I will be coming along to the group to represent the Chief Executive's office and to see if I can help in any way. I know the Chief Executive is looking forward to getting the report and will consider it with great interest. There is pressure from the Department of Health for us to get this right. They are spending half a billion pounds a year on health service food and they are bringing it under the spotlight. New national menu standards are to be introduced and we need to be ahead of the game. I confess it is not a topic I have much of a personal interest in. However, I wonder if I might mention – confidentially – the possibility that we should bring on board Cosmosis, the company undertaking the entrance atrium development. I understand there will be a couple of new food outlets there to serve staff and visitors. Cosmosis may have ideas about how they could contribute to the provision of food and choice for patients as well. It's just a thought.*

Fiona read through these messages with increasing alarm. This really was going to be a time-consuming and complicated business. Even though the working group was only supposed to produce a preliminary report for the senior management team – perhaps with a few recommendations – she felt more confused than before. And she had very little time to process the different views. She made a note to ask Joanne to work up her ideas and budgetary requirements in a little more detail. She also thought she needed to have a chat with Kevin: was there some more money available for catering; and was this Cosmosis issue 'just a thought', or was that the direction in which management wanted to go? She was intrigued, too, by Sudi's emphasis on the health promotion agenda. One of Fiona's practice development projects was with some of her cancer nursing colleagues who were looking at the nutritional needs of cancer patients. This was a return to the importance of the 'feeding' function of the nurse which she felt had become relatively neglected in the face of more technical or more fashionable demands. It was apparent there were also lots of other issues to think about.

March 26th

Fiona had to find Room G7.3 – a meeting room in the new block. Danny was due to present a paper on the patient research he had been doing to his colleagues in the School of Nursing. He had warned Fiona it was going to be 'a bit academic' but she wanted to be there – partly because she was worried about Danny and wanted to keep an eye on him.

The working group had now met twice and there had been some progress – but this related more to pragmatics than to principles. It was clear that Joanne and Kevin had different ideas about the potential resourcing for any new catering initiatives. Joanne had gone back to the drawing board to come up with some more modest resource proposals. It seemed that any involvement on the part of Cosmosis would have to be minimal because of legal and contractual problems. However, Kevin was still interested in closer long-term links between the catering department and Cosmosis and was trying to get Joanne used to the idea.

When it came to issues of principle, though, things had if anything become more confused. Disagreements were sparked when patient concerns about GM food were first mentioned. Sudi had agreed that the priority for patient food should be safety and nutritional content, but she maintained these judgements must be made on scientific grounds – there was no evidence that GM food was unsafe or unhealthy. The representative from Environmental Health who had come to the first meeting came in strongly behind her on this issue. He felt the conditions of the hospital kitchen were only just adequate (and incidentally that nothing should be planned which didn't involve a food safety audit and upgrade). The hospital was there first and foremost to support and protect people's health. This was essentially the terrain of experts. Food choice was valuable but it was of secondary importance. Choice could only be provided within the framework of professional judgement. 'We cannot', he had said, 'respond to every crank, fad or fashion'. Danny had reacted angrily to this, much to Fiona's surprise. He had accused his colleagues of 'professional arrogance'. We were, he argued, supposed to be moving to a patient-centred Health Service – the values and preferences of patients could not and should not be dismissed. He then appealed to the two patient representatives on the working group. They had endorsed his general sentiment, more than this, one of them had expressed her own doubts abut GM food: 'It's all very well saying it's safe now – but scientists are always having to change their minds on these things. Just look at BSE.'

Since that meeting, Fiona had discovered Danny was an active supporter of the Green Party and devoted a lot of his spare time to community and environmental politics. Although she respected his position, she could not help but worry about him being a destabilising influence on the working group. It would only meet once more before she needed to produce a draft report with some recommendation. This would be considered at the group's final meeting. There just wasn't time for a root and branch debate about health service politics. Entering the room where Danny was going to present his paper, Fiona nodded a greeting to him and sat down to listen. She made notes from time to time and that evening took a few minutes to type them up in order to consolidate them in her mind and add them to her working group box file. These are her notes on Danny's paper:

The old days of professional power and authority have gone. The hospital is a publicly funded service. The range of food available in hospitals should be decided as democratically as possible. Decisions about the purchase and use of food products should be made in accordance with the ethical and political beliefs of the population the hospital serves. Decisions should be open to public scrutiny. Although it is not possible to devise simple voting systems for all decisions it is not necessary either. Research (his research for example) shows the importance and potential of patient involvement. The best available mechanisms for extending democratic decision making should be constructed. This is likely to combine the use of surveys, open meetings, and increased patient representation in all hospital planning and evaluation activities. Loads of stuff on different models and theories of democracy and the use of qualitative research in public consultation . . .

Fiona read through what she had typed. The more she thought about it, the more she felt Danny was hi-jacking the agenda. She felt sure the other members of the working group could form a broad consensus on food quality and on the desirability of extending patient food choice; and that they would be able to make recommendations about resources required as well as other practical implications. Danny, though, was calling for something much more far-reaching and – she could not help but feel – something far outside the remit of the group. After the disagreement at the first meeting she had said something along these lines to Danny. He had replied that radical change must begin somewhere and that the working group was as good a place as any.

She read the notes again a couple of times, trying to decide whether or not to take them seriously, and feeling rather ambivalent towards them. On the one hand, the general line seemed plausible. Public involvement in decision-making could be seen as a worthwhile part of 'Food Choice'. On the other hand, it seemed somewhat impractical and perhaps also questionable in some respects. The impracticality was obvious – could everyone in Billingham really decide on whether or not St Alfred's should use free range eggs? Fiona thought that the line's questionable nature came to light if she were to substitute the word 'medicines' for 'food' in her notes. Should decisions about the use of medicines be made democratically? That didn't seem quite right, but then perhaps the case was different?

April 17th

Fiona was relieved to have handed her working group report over to the Chief Executive. She didn't feel she had done a very good job on it but at least it was finished. On the train home that evening she was looking forward to being able to catch up on a backlog of other jobs. But she was also slightly sorry to have to let go of the work on hospital food just as she had got her teeth into it for the first time. (She had made a conscious effort to try and stop puns coming into her mind when she was thinking about the food policy work, but it hadn't been successful!) She took a copy of the eight-page report from her bag and skimmed through it one more time with a strange mixture of shame and pride. Other people were going to be reading through it – would they be disappointed or impressed?

The final shape and content of the report had actually emerged through a series of compromises. Some working group members had wanted it to be shorter and for it to consist essentially of practical recommendations. Others had pressed for the report to reflect the debates and discussions of the group more fully; these complexities, it was suggested, would be obscured if the group simply presented 'recommendations'. In any case, these people had argued, simply listing recommendations would suggest a consensus that simply hadn't existed. Fiona had managed to negotiate a resolution to this conflict. It had been to divide the report into two. The first part set out some of the background issues and debates and signalled the scope of disagreements. The second part laid out the specific recommendations agreed to by the majority of the group, along with some practical implications of these. After this format had been agreed, relationships amongst the working group members had improved substantially, much to Fiona's surprise and delight. She had, for example, tried to work fairly closely with Danny on the first half of the report – he wanted his point of view to be represented and also for his reservations about specific recommendations to be noted. This was, Fiona had realised, a form of consensus. While they had not been able to achieve consensus about the recommendations themselves, they had achieved a near consensus on how to handle their disagreements. She read again the opening pages of the report:

The discussions of the working group on Food Quality and Choice gave rise to a set of debates and disagreements which we believe are worth reporting here. They provide a background to our recommendations and they illustrate the complexity of the issues involved. Having considered the broader food policy context, we believe these working group debates also reflect more general debates about food and society. One area of disagreement within the group was the extent to which the improvement of food quality and choice should be addressed at a societal level rather than at the level of the hospital; and, in particular, the extent to which hospital food policy should be used as a 'lever' for wider change in society. The majority of members of the working group are sceptical about what they see as the 'politicisation' of something they consider to be a practical question of hospital management. However, there is also some strong dissent from this view. We begin by discussing the debates under four headings – health, confidence, uncertainty and accountability.

Health

> *How far should we think of food as a 'tool for health'? Certainly food safety and the control of food poisoning is essential. Beyond that, however, the question is more controversial. Should food be seen principally through the lens of 'nutrition and health' or through other kinds of lenses? On the one hand, food policy experts argue that 'food is a key factor in the main degenerative diseases and causes of premature death such as heart disease, some cancers, obesity and diabetes' (Lang 2000); and that the European Union should ensure 'EU food policies are conducive to consumers being able to eat a diet which enhances health. Policies at the EU level need to work in harmony with national health promotion policies' (European Parliament 2000). On the other hand, food is about much more than nutrition and health. It is a central plank of our cultural life and plays a number of functions within it: for example, as part of cultural symbolism and identity formation; as a dimension of leisure, aesthetic appreciation and enjoyment; and as an expression of our personal preferences and autonomy (Belasco 1997). It is essential therefore that we recognise that there can be some conflict between nutrition and choice, and that both represent important values and concerns. Some may hold the view that hospitals ought to place a particular emphasis on nutrition. And indeed 'clinical nutrition' is a growing part of our research and development agenda. But it is equally possible to argue that simply because people are in hospital does not mean they should be treated as 'captive' targets for health promotion. They should be entitled to make the same 'unhealthy' choices in hospital as they do elsewhere.*

Confidence

> *It is important that members of the public have confidence in the quality of the food they eat. There is increasing evidence of a 'crisis of confidence' in this area. The experience of Bovine Spongiform Encephalopathy (BSE) and its relationship to Creutzfeld-Jacob Disease (CJD) represent a crystallisation of public concerns. These concerns are very wide-ranging and include: scepticism about the transparency and reliability of scientists and policy makers; and criticisms of the prevailing models of food production and distribution – for example, intensive and industrial-scale farming and the effective monopoly held by a few large supermarket chains. Every week there seems to be an escalation of these concerns in relation to further 'food scares' – the use of novel foods such as GM foodstuffs, the re-cycling of condemned poultry scandal, and the 2001 outbreak of Foot and Mouth disease in the UK after a thirty year break. The hospital needs procedures to respond to food scares, and to confidence problems more generally. It needs to be in a position to responsibly reassure its patients where necessary. However it is essential to note that a lack of public confidence may or may not be rationally grounded. (For example, during the Foot and Mouth outbreak a number of consumers stopped eating food products despite assurances that there was no risk to human health from the disease.) Effective 'confidence building measures' must take public concerns seriously whatever their basis. We have to strike a balance between lending credence to*

unfounded public anxieties on the one hand, and treating these fears with due respect on the other.

Uncertainty

It is essential to acknowledge that uncertainty exists in relation to a number of food safety and nutritional matters. Once again, the BSE crisis is the best known exemplar of these uncertainties. The working group was divided as to the depth and breadth of this uncertainty and as to its implications. For example, several members were satisfied with the sort of brief and blanket reassurance provided by the Food Standards Agency with regard to GM foods: 'All GM foods approved for use in the UK have been assessed by independent experts as being as safe as their non-GM counterparts' (Food Standards Agency 2000).

Other members felt that this kind of approach was misleading and possibly counterproductive in its failure to acknowledge the possibility of scientific uncertainty and disagreement – especially in the light of widespread access to more critical perspectives on the safety of foods including novel foods (e.g. Hird 2000). The hospital must recognise that the climate has changed in relation to scientific and medical authority and that the population it serves will not necessarily accept authoritative-sounding reassurances about food matters. Instead we must be ready to provide more nuanced accounts of science and to enter into dialogue about scientific controversies.

Accountability

The management and staff of the hospital are accountable both to the NHS and to the population they serve. We must be ready to explain and defend our policies on food quality and choice. It follows from this that such policies – especially where they become the subject of concern – should be available for public scrutiny. It also follows that both the policies themselves, and the processes by which they are made, should be relatively transparent, and that ideally there is some 'consumer involvement' in policy making (European Parliament 2000). Beyond this, the working group encompassed very different opinions as to the desirability of greater public participation in the making of policy. The majority view, however, was that the legal and ethical obligations of NHS staff require that decision making is essentially done by those staff who are directly accountable for such decisions, and on the basis of the best scientific, medical and professional opinion. These facts severely circumscribe the extent to which wider participation is feasible or justifiable. Against this was a minority view that respect for public opinion requires not only that the public is consulted but also that, insofar as it is possible, decision making should be more equally shared between professionals and the populations they serve.

The train was slowing for her home station so Fiona quickly perused the group's main recommendations: the safety audit; the enhanced menu scheme; the nutritional guidelines; the review of the distribution procedures; the proposal for short written policies on areas of 'food controversy'; a 'light' evaluation strategy for the proposed changes; the cost implications. The whole thing was now out of her hands. She smiled to herself – everything was going to be decided by the Chief Executive's office now in any case. They will look at the report, but will do whatever they want to do.

Power and health promotion ethics

Fiona Haddon's experiences suggest a number of lessons not only for under-standing food policy but also for health promotion ethics in general. In the remainder of this chapter we wish to draw out some of these lessons by reflecting on aspects of the case study in relation to the discussions of power and informed choice with which we began.

It is clear that the members of Fiona's working group found themselves in the midst of a complex system of power relations. Even if they could have agreed what ought to be done, they simply did not have the power to implement their ideas. Changing patterns of food quality and choice – just within the relative confines of a single institution – requires action at a number of levels and in a range of spheres. Further, any possible action has ramifications which spread in every direction. Within the hospital alone, action has implications for a wide range of employees and for the use and control of budgets. None of these things can be changed without the active co-operation of powerful people as well as alterations to the structures and cultures through which power is transmitted. Considered more globally, making changes to food quality and choice has implications not only for public health but also for the economy – for businesses such as retailing, agriculture, transport and distribution and so on. Tracing the lines of power which collectively determine existing patterns of food quality and choice would be an almost impossible conceptual and empirical task. How and where to intervene in order to change these patterns would pose a huge challenge. Would-be health promoters with an interest in food safety and nutrition have to set their efforts within this complex context of causal and power relations. They need also to be ready to see their ideas defeated, or at least compromised, because of a relative lack of power.

However, the case study also suggests there are a number of reasons to be pleased that health promoters may lack power. As we have made clear elsewhere, people value other things and not simply 'health'. Food is an example of some-thing which has relevance and value for both health and non-health reasons. Even if we were to concentrate on ethical issues in food production and con-sumption we would have to look beyond questions of human health. There are important issues about the responsibilities of human beings for the ecosystem in general, and for animal welfare in particular. For many people, these are of much more profound ethical significance than the direct effects of food on human health. What is more, people value food choice in itself as well as for the different values they associate with food. Here, then, as elsewhere, health promoters have to be ready to see health not only in a complex power context but also in a complex value context. To see the truth of this we only have to conduct a simple 'thought experiment'.

Imagine that a group of health promoters 'armed' with the best available knowledge concerning food safety and nutritional disease prevention had the power magically to change the nation's diet. In this fairy tale scenario we might pretend, for example, that they could put something in the water which entirely transformed people's food preferences so that everyone switched to an optimum 'healthy diet'. We would also have to pretend that there was a sufficient supply of suitable good quality food. To focus the issue further we could even make believe that the health promoters' knowledge was absolutely guaranteed (in practice, of course, the lack of any such guarantee is a major reason to be distrustful of expert power). Under these imaginary circumstances would we be happy with these hypothetical health promoters exercising their magical powers?

We suggest that there are good ethical reasons to be most unhappy. Our reasons correspond to the 'consequence-based' and 'rule-based' arguments for and against health promotion that we have rehearsed before. First, we would need to know the total 'side effects' of the health promoters' magic powers. What, for example, might the effects be on animal welfare or, perhaps, on the welfare of farmers? It is quite possible that although the powers have (by definition) beneficial health consequences, their effects considered overall, and taking into account the whole range of valuable things, would be harmful. Myths and fairy tales are full of stories about the unintended and harmful side-effects of magic. Second, this use of magic power entirely fails to respect the choices and autonomy of the population. Even if we might over time come to prefer cabbage to chocolate, say, it does not follow that prior to our change of preference, we would be happy to have this change *forced* upon us. Indeed we are most likely to regard it as an unethical interference in our freedom.

What we are showing here is that there is no point in simply replacing relatively powerless health promoters with relatively powerful ones. Health promoters, just like everyone else, need to 'earn' any influence they have on others if that influence is to be legitimate in an ethical sense. Replacing one system of blind power with another, even where the latter is apparently well meaning, does not in itself alter the ethical shape of things. What matters, ethically speaking, is both the legitimacy, and the responsible use, of power. If health promoters are to build a professional ethic, they need to be critically reflective not only about the power exercised over them, but also about the power they exercise over others. The power hierarchies of the hospital circumscribe the scope of action of Fiona's working group. But the actions of the working group potentially affect the actions and choices of patients. These power relations require health promoters to work with others. To oversimplify, health promoters have to be able to understand and work with the values and the priorities of both 'policy makers' and 'the public'; and they have to be ready, where they think appropriate, to challenge both their own use of power and its exercise by others.

Partly this is simply reiterating our comments at the beginning of the chapter to the effect that health promotion agency transcends the agency of health promoters. The 'accomplishment' of health promotion depends on the involvement of a wide range of agencies. However, we also wish to stress the potential dangers of unreflective and unchallenged health promotion agency. We do so because the hypothetical health promoters with the magic powers we described above are not perhaps quite as much of a fairy tale as they seem. There are a growing number of critiques of the ways in which the languages and practices (or 'discourses') of health promotion have a powerful shaping effect on the ways in which people think and act. (See, for example, Bunton, Nettleton & Burrows 1995). For example, when it comes to food choice, individuals are increasingly making their choices in the light of concerns about health and disease, fitness, or body shape. Further, they are increasingly likely to feel guilty if they do not do so. Health promotion has powerful effects which cannot be represented through the simple deliberate or direct constraining of client autonomy on the part of health promoters. The much more subtle and indirect effects of health promotion discourses are nevertheless both real and pervasive. The worry here is that health promoters may be, albeit unwittingly, party to the growing medicalisation of life. The extent to which the consequences of these processes are negative is a matter of debate. They are, however, an example of health promotion power because they have the effect of shaping individual autonomy – of reinforcing certain values and ways of thinking and undermining others.

In the case of Fiona's working group, for example, there was the question of how far to reform the hospital's food policy by treating food as a 'tool for health'. Although one hospital's approach to this question will obviously not set the whole climate, it is a part of a climate-shaping process. Making a stronger equation between food and health may or may not be a good thing (that is not our central focus here) but it certainly makes a difference to the power relations within the hospital, and to the experiences and choices of patients.

Who decides what to do?

The case study also clearly illustrates that the answer to the question, 'Who decides?' is extremely complex. Not everything that happens is necessarily the result of particular decisions. Some things are 'side-effects' of particular decisions and actions, or are the result of the unintended and unforeseeable interactions between different actions. However, even if we only concentrate on deliberate decisions, there are many of these which determine the quality and choice of food in the hospital. As we made clear at the start of this chapter, it is important to recognise this complexity if we want to ask – and this is one of the questions that proved so controversial for the working group – 'Who *ought* to decide'? Not everyone is equally well placed to contribute to the decision making; and not everyone can be held equally responsible for decisions. We will say a few more words about each of these points.

As Fiona's experience illustrates, there are variations in both power and expertise; although in both cases the nature and the implications of these variations are contestable. Some people might want to confine the relevant expertise to those with appropriate scientific or professional backgrounds. Others would ascribe expertise more widely and recognise different kinds of expertise relevant to the issue being considered. Similarly the distribution of power is contestable. Patients looked at from one point of view – as vulnerable individuals in the hospital 'machine' – are perhaps relatively powerless. Considered, though, as organised groups of 'consumers', they may be able to achieve substantial power. In other words, the relative potential of different agents to contribute to decisions is itself a controversial matter. There is certainly some scope to spread the net of decision-making more widely than is often the case.

Yet this possibility – the possibility of including more people in decision making – does not deal with the second of the two points above. Is it feasible or fair to 'share out' responsibility for decision-making as well as to try and share out power? And, if not, doesn't this limit the real potential for power sharing? This was perhaps the central point of tension between Danny and other members of the working group. The majority of the working group felt that the systems of accountability in which the hospital management and staff worked meant that they ultimately had to take responsibility for the decisions made and, therefore, that it was they who had to take them. We have come up once more against the limits of informed choice in health promotion. We argued at the start of this chapter that the idea of informed choice does not really make sense in the context of populations. There has to be some judgement about which of the things the different members of a population might choose will actually be provided. And some specific people have to make those judgements (Crisp, Hope & Ebbs 1996).

However, we should stress again that whilst there cannot be a 'blanket solution' of giving all potentially affected parties the opportunity to participate in one mass process of 'informed choice'; this does not mean that the principles underlying informed choice can be abandoned in health promotion. Indeed, we suggest the opposite is so. If individuals are important, then populations are important. If respecting people's values and choices is important when making decisions that affect single individuals, we should respect people's values and choices when making decisions which affect many individuals. We may have to be imaginative in constructing the procedures for informing and consulting with groups. We may need to be careful about interpreting, and cautious about implementing, 'the wishes of the group'. We cannot, though, drop the principles simply because their application is challenging. In practice, what health promoters can realistically support is a whole complex of separate informed choices. For example, individual patients can be encouraged to make informed choices about what they choose to eat. Hospital staff can be supported to make informed choices about what range of foods to supply. The local population can be enabled to express informed choices about hospital food policies.

Power hierarchies are pervasive. However much health promoters seek to empower their clients, there will always be power imbalances in decision-making. Yet it does not follow from this fact that there is no point in cultivating and respecting client autonomy, or in clients participating in reaching decisions related to the promotion of health. Indeed, both the substantive soundness and the ethical defensibility of health promotion interventions is optimised by full client participation. Unless health promoters attach a high priority to building these processes of participation they will be ethically negligent. However, as we have also discussed, they will be equally negligent if they seek to simply 'off load' their own professional responsibilities for choices onto their clients.

Section Three
Towards Ethically Defensible Health Promotion

Chapter 7
Codes and Guidelines:
Can They Help Health Promoters?

Introduction

One of the most visible ways in which practitioners – or those representing them – show an interest in ethics is through developing and publishing codes of conduct. These, together with related guidelines, seem to represent an important ethical reference point for those working in particular occupational or professional fields.

In the field of health care, practitioners (or their representatives) see codes and guidelines as ways of declaring the value of their work; of setting out responsibilities in relation to clients or patients; and of making clear what expectations a profession or occupation has of its members (UKCC 1996). From this, codes can also be seen as contributing to prospective or retrospective ethical justification of a particular activity or intervention (Society of Health Education & Health Promotion Specialists 1998).

This list of claims made for codes and guidelines has been drawn directly from publications of two organisations concerned with health promotion and its ethical dimensions: the United Kingdom Central Council for Nursing, Midwifery and Health Visiting (UKCC); and the Society of Health Education and Health Promotion Specialists (SHEPS). At first sight, the claims seem to be both noble and practical. Surely it must be useful to be able to refer to something that can contribute to ethical justification or defence; or that can set standards and establish responsibilities?

But these claims are also ambitious ones. To what extent can codes and guidelines actually accomplish the things claimed for them? Can they be of help to health promoters? In this chapter, we consider this question through an exploration of the codes and related guidelines produced by the two organisations mentioned – the UKCC and SHEPS (UKCC 1992, SHEPS 1997b). These organisations reflect the distinction we have made throughout the book between, on the one hand, health promoters, and on the other, health promotion specialists. The UKCC is the regulatory body responsible for the standards of the professions of nursing, midwifery and health visiting (UKCC

1992).[4] These professions have a central role to play in the promotion of health. Many of their members are active health promoters (arguably all of them should be). By focusing on the UKCC code, we are obviously not suggesting that nurses, midwives and health visitors are the only sorts of professionals who are health promoters. Rather we are treating the code and guidelines for nursing, midwifery and health visiting professionals as emblematic of the problems and possibilities attached to the work of health promoters. And as our primary concern is with the occupational field of health promotion, it is also important to consider the code and related guidelines, developed by SHEPS, for the health promotion specialist.

What are codes and guidelines?

We have already begun to answer this question by pointing to their supposed functions in establishing standards and making explicit responsibilities towards patients or clients.[5] These in turn are likely to support the 'justification' and 'defence' functions of codes and guidelines. However, it is worth looking at the two codes we have chosen to see what they contain and how they present themselves in a little more detail.

Each of these codes follows the 'classic' format for such documents. They both begin with a short preamble, setting out in general the expectations required of those 'governed' by them: 'Each registered nurse, midwife and health visitor shall act ... (UKCC); and 'The duties of the Health Education/ Health Promotion Specialist are based on ...' (SHEPS). This general statement is followed by a series of specific duties or responsibilities: 'As a registered nurse, midwife or health visitor, you are personally accountable for your practice and, in the exercise of your professional accountability, must ...' (UKCC); and 'By taking out membership of the Society of Health Education and Health Promotion Specialists practitioners have ... [certain duties] ... These duties place the following responsibilities on health promoters ...'. (The SHEPS code actually begins with principles of practice from which the central duties and responsibilities cited are presumably derived. And in talking about the responsibilities of 'health promoters', the code is actually referring to what we label as 'health promotion specialists'.)

---

[4] Following legislation, the UKCC was scheduled to be replaced by the new Nursing and Midwifery Council in September 2001. The UKCC was reviewing its Code of Conduct and Guidelines for Professional Practice with the intention of recommending the results of this review to the new Council on the latter's formation. At the time of writing, the results of this review are not known.

[5] Although cumbersome, we will talk about both 'patients' and 'clients' in this chapter. While many in nursing and related professions most naturally speak of the people they work with as 'patients', some refer to them as 'clients'. This might also be the most natural term for those working as health promotion specialists.

UKCC Code of Conduct

Each registered nurse, midwife and health visitor shall act, at all times, in such a manner as to:

- **safeguard and promote the interests of individual patients and clients;**
- **serve the interests of society;**
- **justify public trust and confidence and**
- **uphold and enhance the good standing and reputation of the professions.**

As a registered nurse, midwife or health visitor, you are personally accountable for your practice and, in the exercise of your professional accountability, must:

1 act always in such a manner as to promote and safeguard the interests and well-being of patients and clients;
2 ensure that no action or omission on your part, or within your sphere of responsibility, is detrimental to the interests, conditions or safety of patients and clients;
3 maintain and improve your professional knowledge and competence;
4 acknowledge any limitations in your knowledge and competence and decline any duties or responsibilities unless able to perform them in a safe and skilled manner;
5 work in an open and co-operative manner with patients, clients and their families, foster their independence and recognise and respect their involvement in the planning and delivery of care;
6 work in a collaborative and co-operative manner with health care professionals and others involved in providing care, and recognise and respect their particular contributions within the care team;
7 recognise and respect the uniqueness and dignity of each patient and client, and respond to their need for care, irrespective of their ethnic origin, religious beliefs, personal attributes, the nature of their health problems or any other factor;
8 report to an appropriate person or authority, at the earliest possible time, any conscientious objection which may be relevant to your professional practice;
9 avoid any abuse of your privileged relationship with patients and clients and of the privileged access allowed to their person, property, residence or workplace;
10 protect all confidential information concerning patients and clients obtained in the course of professional practice and make disclosures only with consent, where required by the order of a court or where you can justify disclosure in the wider public interest;
11 report to an appropriate person or authority, having regard to the physical, psychological and social effects on patients and clients, any circumstances in the environment of care which could jeopardise standards of practice;
12 report to an appropriate person or authority any circumstances in which safe and appropriate care for patients and clients cannot be provided;
13 report to an appropriate person or authority where it appears that the health or safety of colleagues is at risk, as such circumstances may compromise standards of practice and care;
14 assist professional colleagues, in the context of your own knowledge, experience and sphere of responsibility, to develop their professional competence, and assist others in the care team, including informal carers, to contribute safely and to a degree appropriate to their roles;
15 refuse any gift, favour or hospitality from patients or clients currently in your care which might be interpreted as seeking to exert influence to obtain preferential consideration and
16 ensure that your registration status is not used in the promotion of commercial products or services, declare any financial or other interests in relevant organisations providing such goods or services and ensure that your professional judgement is not influenced by any commercial considerations.

Notice to all Registered Nurses, Midwives and Health Visitors

This Code of Professional Conduct for the Nurse, Midwife and Health Visitor is issued to all registered nurses, midwives and health visitors by the United Kingdom Central Council for Nursing, Midwifery and Health Visiting. The Council is the regulatory body responsible for the standards of these professions and it requires members of the professions to practise and conduct themselves within the standards and framework provided by the Code.

The Council's Code is kept under review and any recommendations for change and improvement would be welcomed and should be addressed to the:

Registrar and Chief Executive
United Kingdom Central Council
for Nursing, Midwifery and Health Visiting
23 Portland Place
London W1N 3AF

SHEPS Code of Conduct

PRINCIPLES OF PRACTICE AND CODE OF PROFESSIONAL CONDUCT FOR HEALTH EDUCATION & PROMOTION SPECIALISTS

July 1997

The Principles of Practice and Code of Conduct should be used to guide the work of Health Education and Promotion Specialists and others working in the fields of health education, health promotion and public health. The Principles of Practice and Code of Conduct reflect the values expressed in the WHO Health For All Strategy, the Ottawa Charter and Agenda 21.

The Society defines Health Promotion as follows:

'Health promotion is any activity that promotes health. Health promotion is achieved through activity focused on the social, economic and environmental determinants of health'

Health promotion includes health education which the Society defines as:

'Activity intended to inform and empower people so that they can make high quality decisions about health issues'

PRINCIPLES OF PRACTICE

The following Principles of Practice constitute the basis of the Code of Professional Conduct. Any member of the Society of Health Education and Promotion Specialists who is deemed by the Society to have contravened any of the following principles or duties of the Code will be subject to disciplinary action which may result in expulsion from the Society.

The duties of the Health Education/Health Promotion Specialist are based on fundamental ethical and professional principles relating to the maximisation of health.

Relationship to Client/Recipient

1   Adequate needs assessment, consultation with and involvement of the client or target group is essential to the effective planning, implementation and reviewing of Health promotion activities.
2   The promotion of self esteem and autonomy amongst client groups/recipients should be an underlying principle of all health promotion practice.
3   Health promotion should encourage people to value others whatever their gender, age, race, class, religion, culture, sexuality, ability or health status, and attempt to counter prejudice and discrimination wherever it occurs.

Social and Environmental Influences

4   Health promotion programmes should be relevant and sensitive to the nature of the intended client group – for example the social, economic and cultural framework of the group.
5   Health promotion work should include recognition of and action focused on the social, economic and environmental determinants of health.
6   Health promotion work should aim to empower and enable people to exercise informed choice and influence structures and systems that have an impact on health.
7   Health promotion programmes which focus on specified issues should always be set in the wider political, social, economic, geographical, psychological and environmental context which has a bearing on health.
8   The sustainability of health promotion interventions needs to be considered within the context of the aims of any programme of activity. Health promotion interventions should aim to have a positive impact on both the immediate recipients and future generations of people.

Health Promotion Practice

A   An aim of health promotion practice is to bring about change in the social and economic environment to improve health and to reduce or eliminate inequalities in health at a local, national and international level.
B   Appropriate research and evaluation is an essential component of health promotion activity. Practitioners should endeavour to disseminate results and findings.
C   Practitioners have a responsibility for ensuring an accurate and appropriate information flow between the public, professionals, local and national agencies, and for taking the initiative and responding accordingly.
D   Practitioners will endeavour to provide services or information that they have at their disposal that would, in the light of current theory and/or evidence, maintain and promote health. They will endeavour to keep their knowledge of current developments in health promotion up to date.
E   Practitioners will have due regard to the confidentiality of information to which they have access, bearing in mind the requirements of the law.
F   Health promotion work should encourage all services and organisations to develop their health promotion role and to adopt the above principles of practice.

G   Health promotion activity is by its nature a collaborative endeavour. Practitioners should seek to actively collaborate with colleagues and others to promote health.
H   The methods and process of health promotion should be health promoting.

CODE OF PROFESSIONAL CONDUCT

By taking out membership of The Society of Health Education and Health Promotion Specialists practitioners have a:

i)   duty to care
ii)   duty to be fair
iii) duty to respect personal and group rights
iv) duty to avoid harm
v)   duty to respect confidentiality
vi) duty to report

These duties place the following responsibilities on health promoters:

1   not to harm people and/or colleagues by wilful deception or by knowingly misinforming on health matters;
2   not to harm people and/or colleagues by involving them in health promotion activities – nor provide materials, resources or experiences – which are damaging or inappropriate;
3   not knowingly to participate in health promotion activities for which the practitioner is not adequately trained or competent;

4   not to discriminate by any act or omission against anyone on the basis of gender, age, race, class, religion, culture, sexuality, disability or health status;
5   not to exploit any individual, group or employer with the primary purpose of personal gain or satisfaction;
6   not to engage in competition for services which would lead to a negative impact on individual, group or community health;
7   not to be involved in the provision of services designed solely to meet the demands of income generation or other subsidiary goals at the expense of meeting demonstrable health needs;
8   not to wilfully withhold available services or information needed by people to make health choices;
9   not to breach confidentiality or invade personal privacy;
10 not to compromise professional credibility by engaging in inappropriate collaboration with commercial enterprises or other organisations whose objectives are incompatible with health promotion principles and practice;
11 not to take any deliberate unjustifiable action which may bring members into disrepute or undermine their position; this does not preclude constructive professional criticism.

In each case, the duties or responsibilities are framed within a single sentence. How is it possible for one sentence to adequately give reasonable direction on ethical matters where we have consistently argued that at both theoretical and practical levels, their nature is enormously complex? The simple answer – and one which the code-makers themselves would probably agree with – is that it can't. So the final element of the 'classic' structure of codes is that they are supported by more detailed supplementary guidance, appearing in other places. In the case of the UKCC code, a number of further documents provide this guidance, including 'Guidelines for Professional Practice' (UKCC 1996). For the SHEPS code, guidance comes in the form of a series of briefing papers (SHEPS 1998). So article 16 of the UKCC code states that practitioners should:

'Ensure that your registration status is not used in the promotion of commercial products or services, declare any financial or other interests in relevant organisations providing such goods or services and ensure that your professional judgement is not influenced by any commercial considerations...' (UKCC 1992).

Pages 31–33 of the 'Guidelines for Professional Practice' cover the subject of advertising and sponsorship and aim to provide substantially greater guidance on these issues than the single sentence of the code allows.

Equally, article seven of the SHEPS code requires health promotion specialists:

> 'Not to be involved in the provision of services designed solely to meet the demands of income generation or other subsidiary goals at the expense of meeting demonstrable health needs...' (SHEPS 1997b).

And again, much more guidance than this one sentence can give is provided in a briefing paper on the subject of income generation (SHEPS 1998).

This description of these codes and related documents suggests a way of understanding the nature of, and relationship between, codes of conduct and guidelines for practice. According to the 'classic' format against which the two examples we are thinking about seem to have been constructed, codes express more or less general obligations or responsibilities on the part of practitioners. It is clear, aside of anything else, that the language used by each code understands what it says to be binding – if the code is to be adhered to these obligations *must* be met:

> 'Each registered nurse, midwife and health visitor *shall act, at all times*, in such a manner...' (UKCC code, our emphasis).

> 'The following Principles of Practice constitute the basis of the Code of Professional Conduct. Any member ... who is deemed by the Society to have *contravened any of the following principles or duties of the Code will be subject to disciplinary action which may result in expulsion from the Society...*' (SHEPS code, our emphasis).

Guidelines supply much greater detail. But it is worth noting that often guideline writers move to less directive and more conditional language, as they give advice on what might be implied by the obligations contained in the code. For example, article 10 of the UKCC code states that practitioners must:

> 'Protect all confidential information concerning patients and clients obtained in the course of professional practice and make disclosures only with consent, where required by the order of a court or where you can justify disclosure in the wider public interest...' (UKCC 1992).

But the related guidance notes that continuing consent to exchanges of information (possibly relatively quite minor) between different health care staff may be impractical and argues that only general awareness of such exchanges may be required by the patient or client. How general this awareness is, and how this is conveyed to the client or patient, is hard to specify and thus difficult to frame as a strict obligation. Besides, if attempts were made to do this, it would fail to allow the possibility of professional discretion. Not surprisingly then, more extensive guidelines yield more possible courses of action. Which one of these is taken can be allowed to the individual (or she or he may take another one altogether). Someone may have accepted the obligation of not overdrawing on their bank account each month, but this can be done in a number of ways (much less on phone bills, a bit less on food). Equally, we may have a definitive obligation to protect confidentiality and ensure consent, but this may be achieved through a variety of methods. If codes place definitive obligations on practitioners, guidelines offer support on how those obligations can be fulfilled.

These requirements and suggestions serve the purpose of clarifying the nature of three different sets of relationships: the relationships between individual practitioners and their patients or clients; the much more general relationship between a profession or occupation and the public it is supposed to be serving; and the relationship between practitioners within the same occupation or profession.

Much of what is contained in codes of ethics might be thought of as declarations of intent. (Some of the discussion that follows concentrates on codes where these declarations are in sharper focus, although we have emphasised the reciprocal nature of the relationship between codes and guidelines). In the context of the practitioner-patient relationship, for example, a code of conduct is an attempt to promote trust through establishing expectations. If we seek the help of a nurse, say, then we can expect that he or she will, among other things, 'promote and safeguard [our] interests and well-being': 'ensure that no action or omission [on her or his part] is detrimental to [our] interests, condition or safety'; and 'recognise and respect [our] uniqueness and dignity...' (all of these are obligations taken at random from the UKCC code). Of course, we probably won't be going to a nurse and saying explicitly that this is what we expect from her or his dealings with us; and equally she or he will probably not be presenting us with the list of obligations expressed in the code at our first meeting and saying, 'Look – you can trust me!' But this is perhaps the point. Generally we believe we can trust nurses to try and look after our welfare and so on. Our trust is usually implicit, but if we wanted to, we could check on the rationale for it through reference to the code.

Part of the reason why we have the general belief of trust that we do in nurses relates to a second purpose of codes – that of representing a profession to its public. Codes are representations by a given profession or occupation of its concern to guarantee standards. If you choose, or are obliged, to seek the help of the profession of nursing, for example; then *the profession* is saying that this is what you have a right to expect from any one of its members. One of the expectations that might follow from the UKCC code, as we have said, is that the nurse will promote our interests and well-being. We have this expectation – even if only implicitly – of the nurse who advises us on a healthier diet just before we are discharged from hospital; of the nurse at the general practice who immunises our child; and indeed of any other nurse with whom we come into contact.

Sometimes, of course, our expectations, and thus our trust, are misplaced. We can probably all think of occasions when we haven't been treated as we would think appropriate by health care professionals. Some of these, perhaps, have been caused by lack of time, or other pressures. In other words, trust has not been deliberately abused. In some cases, however, deliberate abuse of trust is present; and in the worst of these we can be shocked by both the degree of abuse and its consequences – the case of the paediatric nurse Beverley Allitt, for example, convicted of murdering children on the Grantham hospital ward where she worked.

This moves us to the third kind of relationship clarified by codes – the relationship between members of the same profession or occupation. All members of the profession of nursing, have in at least one respect a particular kind of relationship with each other – they are all bound by the UKCC code. But as Beverley Allitt and other cases show, the code cannot guarantee that trust is warranted. Surely almost all nurses, though, would not want to share a relationship with Beverley Allitt. This is not least because if we thought that the nurse immunising our child was in any relevant respect like Beverley Allitt, we would not be having the child immunised by that nurse. But the point is that the nurse doing the immunisation no longer shares a relationship with Beverley Allitt because – by virtue of what the latter did – she has been struck off the register of nurses (as well as being removed from society). So in the case of nurses, a further part of the relationship they share with each other is that they can be removed from their profession (removed from the professional register) if they fail to live up to its expectations to the extent that they breach its code (Pyne 1995). Nurses are bound in expectations of trust to one another; and individual nurses and the corporate nursing body are bound in relationships of trust with the patients and public they serve.

All this suggests that – at least in the case of nursing – the code of conduct in conjunction with the tools for professional regulation (in particular, the professional register) provides an incentive for practitioners in this area to take obligations seriously and behave ethically. We hope that nurses will do this because they freely want to and because the obligations correspond with their personal values and motivations. We may be more certain that they will because if they don't, personal and career consequences are potentially calamitous. Some nurses will still fail in their obligations and deliberately abuse trust; but in the context of the regulatory mechanisms that exist, they will cease to be people who we subsequently need to trust in the same way.

We have so far related the purpose of the UKCC code of conduct to establishing, governing and regulating relationships between practitioners and patients, professions and public. At least some of the practical power it (and its associated guidelines) possess is because adherence to the code is required in order for a nurse, midwife or health visitor to continue to practise. Being able to work in one or other of these capacities is contingent on registration (following prescribed training); and maintaining registration is equally contingent on not breaching the code. The code for health promotion specialists – the SHEPS code – provides a contrast.

The SHEPS code is expressed as much in 'musts' as that of the UKCC. The difference is that the language of 'must' is arguably more appropriate in the case of the UKCC because the 'musts' are properly enforceable for nurses, midwives and health visitors; whereas for health promotion specialists they are not (or at least not in terms of statutory professional regulation). We are however simply using 'must' to mean 'required by adherence to the professional code' irrespective of whether this requirement is professionally enforced.

The whole occupational context of the health promotion specialist is less structured and regulated. While it can certainly be argued that the job of health promotion specialist requires particular (and valuable) kinds of skills and expertise, uniform and mandatory training does not exist. A growing number of higher education institutions offer undergraduate and postgraduate programmes in health promotion, but the courses on offer differ widely in terms of both approach and content (Bremner 1994, Cotter 1994). Further, there is no requirement on someone applying for, or even working in, a health promotion specialist post actually to have undertaken either an undergraduate or a post-graduate course. Essentially, anyone has the potential to practise as a health promotion specialist (although obviously employers (as well as SHEPS) have ideas about the kinds of skills and backgrounds required in order to do the job effectively). The 'register' of health promotion specialists (SHEPS 1991) is informal and appearance on it is a voluntary decision. If a specialist breaches the code of conduct, sanctions would amount only to reprimand by SHEPS or possibly withdrawal of membership if the person breaching the code is a Society member. But this need not have any effect on the person's status as a practising health promotion specialist because there is no fixed relationship between either registration or membership and capacity to practice. Anyone can do so – and they can continue to do so even if they breach the code.

Does all this mean that we have reason to trust health promotion specialists less than we trust nurses, midwives and health visitors? One possible response to this question is that we don't, as a matter of fact, need to trust health promotion specialists as much as we do nurses, midwives and health visitors. In general, those bound by the UKCC code are likely to be dealing with individual patients or clients in actually or potentially difficult or threatening situations. Think, for example, of the nurse looking after the intensive care patient, or the midwife involved in a difficult childbirth. On the other hand health promotion specialists work in much less acute situations and usually not directly with individuals in need. Their role is much more one of co-ordination and facilitation of health promotion work by other occupational or professional groups. Surely there is less need to trust the health promotion specialist engaged in training health promoters to be more effective in smoking prevention than there is to trust the intensive care nurse looking after the critically ill patient (administering drugs, monitoring and maintaining vital signs and so on)?

This is a dubious position for three reasons. First, its implication is that some kinds of health and health care work are less important than others. If we feel the need to trust the intensive care nurse, more than the need to trust the health promotion specialist, aren't we in danger of attaching less significance to the health promotion specialist's work? Of course, it is possible to have different degrees of trust in different situations. We have a fairly casual degree of trust in the person who sells us a paper at the newsagent that it will be what we expect and that they will give us the right change. We have (or more precisely need to have) rather firmer trust in the plumber who is fixing our central heating that they will get it right, particularly if the breakdown has happened in the middle of winter. These different degrees do not relate simply to the fact that in both cases financial transactions of greater or lesser amounts are taking place. They relate much more centrally to the value of the separate goods involved. Generally speaking, our lives are not going to be much affected if our change at the newsagent is a little bit short, or even if we get the wrong paper. However, if our central heating in winter time remains unfixed, then we will sharply feel the lack of this particular good.

But the point about our differently trusting those who supply us with different goods is simply that the goods are different, and so different levels of trust are appropriate. In the case of the intensive care nurse and the health promotion specialist, they are both engaged in promoting broadly the same good of health (whether understood as the 'absence of disease' or more holistically).

Also, both the specialist and the health promoter are often engaged together in a shared enterprise. If we suggest there is less importance to be attached to some parts of this enterprise than others, then this mitigates against the shared nature of the enterprise. The enterprise is shared precisely because its different parts are connected more or less directly. The intensive care nurse might be looking after someone recovering from major surgery for heart disease, arguably attributable in part to a lifetime of heavy smoking. It is easy to set out such connections between many health care interventions and in doing so, the lines between them and their effects become much less clear-cut.

Finally, and perhaps most important, we trust (or need to trust) health care workers because we believe (or want to believe) that they will not intentionally subject us to risk or harm in our dealings with them. The health promotion specialist is equally capable of placing people at risk and subjecting them to harm as is the intensive care nurse. The nurse may give the wrong injection or put up the wrong drip and this may have consequences immediately threatening to life. But the specialist who is training practice nurses, say, and who advocates relatively coercive methods to achieve patient compliance in behaviour change is also undertaking action that might result in risk or even harm.

Thus it is hard to argue – at least in a general sense – that the social maintenance of trust is less important in some aspects of health care than in others. Because health care is a shared and connected field; and because the potential for risk and harm is present right the way through health care (including health promotion); it seems wrong to suggest that we need to trust the health promotion specialist (bound by the SHEPS code) less than the nurse, midwife or health visitor as health promoter (bound by the UKCC code). We need to be able to trust both.

To summarise: codes have a function in terms of determining the nature of the relationship between professionals and their patients or clients. More specifically, they enable the former to promote trust and guarantee standards to the latter. They represent the profession or occupation to the wider public, again through their functions of promoting trust and guaranteeing standards and through their supporting processes of professional or occupational regulation. They provide guidance to members of the occupation or profession on dealing with ethically difficult situations. And they contribute to establishing the nature of the relationship between members of the profession, and bind professions or occupations together through providing justification for that profession or occupation. They do this because their authority is derived from their expression of the purpose of that profession or occupation. The centrality of concern for well-being in the UKCC code fundamentally relates to the belief that nursing's purpose is about protecting and promoting well-being; and equally, in the SHEPS code and principles, the prominence of autonomy reflects the concern of those involved in the specialism that health promotion can only be both effective and a good if it is empowering (Tones & Tilford 1994).

Codes, 'enforcement' and 'the ethical practitioner'

A distinction has been drawn in this chapter between the different contexts in which the separate codes we are discussing operate. This is the distinction in terms of what might be called 'the context of regulation and enforcement'. The UKCC code can be understood as one of a number of mechanisms (together with statutory training and registration) contributing to nursing's strict context of regulation and enforcement. In order to practise as a nurse, a prescribed period of training must be followed: the intending practitioner must apply to be registered as such; and maintaining status as a registered practitioner is dependent on not breaching the code. In contrast, the context of regulation and enforcement in which the health promotion specialist operates is weak, arguably even non-existent. There is no prescribed training: no requirement to register as a practitioner; and therefore no sense in which 'code breach' could result in disciplinary action or removal from the occupation.

As we have said, all this might suggest to some that health promotion specialists, by virtue of the unregulated nature of their occupation, might be less
worthy of trust than nurses. It seems to reflect common sense and our knowledge
of human nature that the presence of regulation and possible sanctions often
causes us to act in certain ways. When I drive into my nearest town, I slow down
as I pass through the built-up area. I hope that my motivation for doing so is out
of a concern for the welfare of pedestrians and other vehicles in this busier place.
But at least part of my motivation is a wish not to get stopped by the police for a
speeding offence. If the possibility of sanctions being applied for acting in a
certain way (speeding) was not present, I may be more likely to drive faster than
my consideration for the welfare of others alone would allow. Equally, we hope
that we can trust nurses because they are motivated by concerns for human
welfare; but we may feel more certain of that trust because we know that if it is
breached, they will be subject to sanctions. In the case of the health promotion
specialist, we might have similar hopes for trust based on their motivations.
However, no reinforcement in the form of sanctions ('official' ones at least) to
particular trustworthy ways of behaving exists here. If I might be more likely to
speed if no rules against speeding are enforced; the health promotion specialist
might be more likely to be untrustworthy in their context of regulation and
enforcement.

Of course, we want to emphasise straight away that our point here is theoretical rather than empirical. In practice, we all know that most people's motivations to ethical occupational action do not rest purely on fears of being
sanctioned! We have argued that we need to trust both nurses and health promotion specialists equally; and we would strongly suggest that in practice, more
often than not, it is reasonable to do so. However if a code 'has teeth' are not
practitioners more inclined to keep to it? And does this not mean that such codes
are a more effective support to professional ethics?

There is an assumption underlying this thought that we want to challenge. The
assumption is this: the fact of enforceability (making sure that rules really *must* be
kept to) ensures that practitioners will behave ethically (that is to say, do what
they *ought*).

We want to emphasise again here that we are only pursuing a line of argument.
We are not making a claim that, empirically speaking, there is a relationship
between the way practitioners regard codes of conduct (with more or less seriousness) and the status of those codes in terms of their enforceability. Such
empirical work would be a task for disciplines such as psychology or sociology.
Our interest is more fundamental; what, in a conceptual sense, is the relationship
between what we *must* do and what we *ought* to do? Our suggestion is that a
code's 'having teeth' is not by itself a guarantee that it is more likely to promote
ethical action. We say this because *must* (the official or legal requirement) is
simply not the same as *ought* (the ethical requirement). If this is acknowledged,
then from an ethical point of view, the nature of the UKCC and the SHEPS codes

becomes much more equivalent. The latter may no longer be seen as the 'poor relation' of the former. The level of enforceability of a code is an indication of its capacity to support 'professional ethics' only if professional ethics is reduced to 'obedience to a code'. But this presupposes that: (a) the contents of a code are the unqualified arbiter of ethics and are immune to ethical critique; (b) the contents of a code, and associated rules and guidelines, can be applied to reality in an unproblematic and 'self-interpreting' way; and (c) that codes encompass all of the dimensions of ethical thought and action. After a few moments' thought it should be clear that none of these presuppositions are realistic.

In this respect codes of ethics are no different from 'the law' in general. Someone striving to be an ethical practitioner needs to understand that laws are not necessarily ethically defensible, and that even where they are following the law, this is not sufficient for ethics – laws still need to be interpreted in ethically responsible ways, and laws provide a partial (not comprehensive) guide to action. (But this analogy with 'the law' also makes it clear that codes of ethics have a function in ethical life. They provide a *prima facie* reason for action, and – given that the practitioner is satisfied that the relevant component of the code is apposite and ethically acceptable – they provide for a degree of predictability and reliability in professional conduct which is, in itself, a valuable element of trust.)

The understanding that *must* is not the same as *ought* begins with the recognition – apparent throughout this book – that health care practices are frequently complex; and relationships between practitioners and their patients or clients often messy and difficult. If practices are complex, and relationships messy, it will sometimes (probably quite often) be the case that more than one reasonable course of action is open to a practitioner. There will be occasions when following the rules of a code of conduct (doing what *must* be done) may not be the right action (what an individual *ought* to do). Consider the following example. A health promotion specialist is approached by the local outlet of a multinational take away food company. The company is offering, with absolutely no strings attached, to provide space in its restaurant for information in support of a 'Say No to Drugs' campaign. More than this, it is offering to pay for the production of this information in a glossy format that would be likely to appeal to the many young people who use the restaurant as a meeting place. It would be impossible for the specialist to pay for such attractive production using conventional funding sources. There is, let us suppose, good reason to believe that the combination of the kind of information, and the location where young people would be encountering it, would contribute to positive awareness – raising of issues around drugs and drug misuse. But the specialist is also aware that this multinational company has a dreadful record on environmental protection and the use of cheap labour in developing countries. What should she do? The SHEPS code of conduct contains a relevant *must:*

'[The health promoter has a duty] not to compromise professional credibility by engaging in inappropriate collaboration with commercial enterprises or other organisations whose objectives are incompatible with health promotion principles and practice . . .' (SHEPS 1997b).

A reasonable interpretation of the situation facing the specialist would be that collaboration is inappropriate (the company's global objectives have nothing to do with health promotion) so that in order to adhere to the code she must not get involved. There will be some who claim that in this case, *ought* is in fact the same as *must*. Rejecting collaboration is the ethical course of action. Yet for others, the issue might be more ambiguous. In saying no to the company's offer, the specialist is also ruling out the possibility of a health promotion intervention that may very well produce benefit in terms of raising young people's awareness. There will be some prepared to argue that what the specialist *ought* to do is to collaborate, despite the *must* exhortation from the code. Whether or not we agree this is not an unreasonable position. (It is important to see that both sides – those advocating that she does not follow the Code and those who wish her to do so – can make recourse to explicitly *ethical* arguments to justify their positions.)

Of course, part of the difficulty stems from the possibility of different interpretations of the intervention and its context (individuals giving more or less weight in their judgement to the record of the company and to the worth of the activity). But this brings us back to the point we are making. To suggest in this example – and, we would argue, in many others – that *must* is the same as *ought* does not pay enough attention to its messy and problematic context. Would we be happy that the specialist was acting ethically if she simply excluded all considerations of context and blindly followed the 'rule' laid down by the Code? If she did, her stance might remind us of Mr T – the 'pure technician' – in Chapter 4. It may be in this case that she reaches the conclusion that *must* and *ought* push in the same direction; but it is in deliberation rather than simply rule-following that this conclusion has ethical relevance.

Regardless of our own personal position in relation to this example (what we would do), we are able to see that others might do (or at least think about doing) differently, and do it with ethical seriousness. It is possible to conceive of situations where the right course of action may not be to adhere to the rules. Two consequences flow from this. First, codes may sometimes prescribe action that some, at least, would regard as 'unethical'. Second, codes may potentially limit practitioners' capacity to deliberate on a situation and decide on a course of action they believe to be ethical.

The first point is self-evident from our discussion so far. The second point requires further explanation. Codes of conduct are designed to be impressive documents, attempting to convey, as we have seen, much about the nature of a profession or occupation: how that profession or occupation wishes to be seen by those using its services; and how the relationship between the profession or occupation and its members should be understood. It might be hard for a practitioner not to feel rather daunted or in awe of a code (and mechanisms related to it, if there are any). She or he might feel that the ethical relevance and importance of her or his work is contained within the code. There will of course, be many occasions where sticking close to the code is in fact the right thing to do. But as we have just seen, there will be other situations of greater ambiguity or difficulty. A practitioner in awe of a code – or simply believing it contains 'all the answers' – may miss such problems or feel that he or she simply doesn't have the capacity themselves to make ethical sense of a particular situation.

A further consideration which should lead us to put codes into perspective is that they simply leave out any reference to so much that is important in health care practice. Much of both the UKCC and the SHEPS codes, if they are examined carefully, is concerned with describing what might be thought of as 'negative duties' – to avoid causing harm, extending beyond the limits of individual competence and so on. What is often missing in them is an emphasis on encouraging the positive human (intellectual or emotional) qualities of the good practitioner. Of course, to some degree this is because specifying what people must not do is easier than specifying what they ought to do, or ought to be like. We can legislate against, say, a bad nurse; but we cannot similarly legislate for the creation of 'good' (caring, compassionate) nurses. The development of such people is through a complex of factors including natural predisposition, appropriate mentoring, sensitive training, encouragement of reflective ability and so on. This kind of development sounds very different to the simple, uncomplicated requirement to adhere to a code of conduct. But from whom would we rather receive health promotion advice? The nurse following a code of conduct based primarily on 'negative duties'; or one developing their capacity to care and to act ethically in the much broader sense we have just indicated?

Conclusion

We have spent some time arguing that codes of ethics have limitations. The right course may not be to follow the rules in a given situation; and certain uses of codes may potentially limit a practitioner's capacity for individual decisions with regard to the ethics of their activity.

To some degree, we have emphasised these limitations because of the tendency of those promoting codes of conduct to overplay their value as tools for ethical support. However, we do not want to suggest that codes and related guidelines have no use. Clearly they do, for reasons enumerated in the first half of this chapter and not least because they offer one means for reflecting on sensitive and ambiguous areas of practice. Codes can be one of the mechanisms for supporting the development of the 'good' practitioner we described above. But there is a need to be aware of the limits to the support codes and guidelines can offer; and, particularly, to be dubious about the view that simply 'following the rules' (or guidelines) is sufficient to make a practitioner ethical. What is needed is an alternative conception of a code of conduct and of the nature of the relationship between that code and the practitioner.

According to one (perhaps simplistic) view, the ethical practitioner is the person who is able to select and apply the 'right' principle or article from the code that governs her or his professional or occupational activity. Here ethics is seen as something that can be applied from the 'outside in' (from the code to the practitioner) (Dawson 1994). But this depends on the code or guidelines always and obviously fitting every practice situation – something which is impossible. It is not just that codes tend to be prescriptive rather than capacity-building, but that they obviously need to be actively interpreted and applied case by case. An alternative – and we suggest more plausible – conception is of ethical judgement as something that moves from the 'inside out' (Dawson 1994). Here, the ethical practitioner is someone who is encouraged to develop their ethical judgement and capacity. This person not only knows that a particular principle or article of a code exists; he or she also understands its sources and knows how to apply it. An important part of this 'knowing how' includes an interest in the bases of ethical conduct and a concern with how it might be possible to lead a good personal and professional life. This is a much more demanding project and codes of conduct are only one part of this project. The last two chapters of this book will explore some of the other components.

Chapter 8
Lessons From Applied Ethics

Introduction

In this book we set out to build an understanding of how values and ethics are fundamental to the field of health promotion, and of how work to promote health might become more sensitive towards, and better able to deal with, the central ethical tensions that define the field. If applied philosophy is understood as the application of philosophical techniques to areas of practical concern, such as health care (Society for Applied Philosophy 2000), then a lot of this book might be seen as an exercise in applied philosophy and applied ethics. Hopefully we have done enough already to convince you that ethics can usefully be applied to health promotion. But the emphasis we have chosen has been upon 'professional ethics' – on reflective practice about the values and ethical dilemmas facing practitioners – we have only really scratched the surface of applied philosophy and ethics. In this chapter we want to reflect on the contribution of applied philosophy and ethics to health promotion. This will provide a means for us to summarise some of the earlier discussions, but, more importantly, we hope it will begin to indicate the huge further potential for applying philosophy to health promotion for those who wish to move beyond the constraints of professional ethics.

The latter half of the chapter will briefly review the ways in which applied ethics – particularly bioethics or health care ethics – is useful to health promoters. We will also reflect a little on some of the historical affinities between health care ethics and health promotion. But first we think it is worth saying something about academic ethics and applied ethics more broadly – are these things not perhaps a waste of time for practitioners faced with the day to day pressures of health work?

Academic ethics – a waste of time?

Ethics is both the name of an academic discipline and the name of its subject matter. Academic ethics is a branch of philosophy concerned with the study of (in a nutshell) what is right or good. It ranges from very abstract theoretical questions about the bases and nature of ethical judgement to more applied concerns with important social questions about, for example, human welfare, social justice, and our duties to other animals or the environment. Like all philosophical subjects it is characterised by continuing disagreements and debates, including disagreements about the nature of the discipline, suitable starting points and how to 'do' ethics. To someone entering the field for the first time, the pervasiveness and depth of these disagreements might well suggest that they are entering a chaotic domain! However as they gain greater familiarity with the texts and discussions they would come to quite the opposite conclusion.

Academic ethics is oriented towards clarification, order and systematic argument. Differences and debates are conspicuous precisely because they are being so carefully mapped and analysed. And part of this mapping function is the careful clarification and elaboration of concepts, assumptions and arguments. Thus even if academic ethics does not offer the health promoter clear procedures for resolving ethical issues it is well suited to helping the health promoter achieve greater clarity about what is at stake in health promotion ethics. Later we will turn to this clarification and mapping function but we must first address a fundamental issue which can 'get in the way' of taking academic ethics seriously in the first place. We can present this issue in the words of a potential sceptic:

> 'In the end is not ethics essentially just a matter of opinion, and given this fact surely no amount of clarification or discussion can make a real difference? In other fields – such as physics or history – there may be a lot of uncertainty and debate, but participants in these debates normally feel that there is some kind of underlying reality about which they are trying to make a judgement. They tend to believe that there are better and worse answers to their questions and if they revise their views it is because they come to see a better answer, an answer that is 'closer to the truth'. When it comes to ethics, people might change their minds about things – and reading or talking about academic ethics might prompt these changes – but this merely results in different views, not better views. When all is said and done it is just opinion B rather than opinion A. The reading and talking is just froth.'

We believe that these concerns deserve to be taken seriously. Anyone studying ethics needs to ask these questions. And those people who are primarily studying ethics as part of their professional education and development are bound to be sceptical. They can do without froth!

Our own view, unsurprisingly, is that academic ethics is of practical relevance, and in particular that there can be a direct connection between the processes of clarifying and discussing on the one hand and the production of better answers on the other. But as we set this view out more fully in what follows we expect our remarks to be examined with a critical and sceptical eye.

Ethical relativism and ethical justification in everyday discourse – two rival currents

The sceptic's remarks which appear above reflect a prominent current in everyday talk about ethics. They express a form of 'ethical relativism' – the view that not only are there different views in ethics but that there are no reliable means of evaluating the relative strengths and weaknesses of these views. There is a broad cluster of factors that underpin this current. People may point to the diversity of ethical beliefs – historically, geographically, or culturally. There is no doubt that the nature and influence of certain important ethical beliefs (e.g. about the status of women or children) shift over time. And it is equally clear that many fundamental ethical beliefs (e.g. about the acceptability of abortion or capital punishment) vary between (and within) cultures and sub-cultures. There is, therefore, what might be called 'practical relativity' about ethics or 'ethical pluralism'. Whilst it is important to see that ethical relativism does not follow from ethical pluralism (you cannot infer 'equally valid' views from the fact of multiple views), it is easy to see how ethical pluralism may incline people in the direction of relativism. For, they will be inclined to say, 'Who can stand outside all of this diversity and make judgements about it?'

For very good reasons people often do not wish to be intolerant or 'judgemental' about other people's views. We wish to treat other people and other cultures with respect. And, finally, we are surely right to exercise some intellectual and ethical humility about our capacity to arbitrate between rival ethical belief systems. Is it not possible that we are wrong? So ethical pluralism, tolerance and a proper humility can incline us in the direction of relativism. This current is so powerful and so ingrained that it is sometimes expressed simply as an unthinking assumption. It is not unusual to hear someone use the phrase 'Well that is a value judgement' to mean 'It is simply relative'.

But there is another equally powerful current in everyday discourse which is manifest in the existence of ethical debate. People normally take their ethical beliefs very seriously indeed. At least with respect to many of these beliefs they do not hold them as if they are just 'a matter of opinion'. Furthermore this seriousness is not just a matter of the intensity with which ethical beliefs are held; it is shown by the fact that people typically seek to *justify* their beliefs to one another.

In televised discussions of capital punishment, for instance, the protagonists will seek to justify their respective positions by advancing *reasons* to support them. If the same people were talking about their preferences for wine they might simply say 'You prefer red wine, I prefer white wine – it is just a question of taste.' But there is no equivalent move in the case of capital punishment. If someone were to say 'You prefer capital punishment, I prefer no capital punishment – it is just a question of taste', this would be barely intelligible. This capital punishment discussion is not about individual taste but is a debate about the best judgement we can make about something. (In the wine example the two parties are talking about themselves, and they are not actually disagreeing about anything. In the capital punishment case they are talking about something external to them both and are disagreeing about it.)

People who work in health promotion, like everyone else, hold certain ethical beliefs sincerely and sometimes passionately. They may, for example, be strongly committed to equal opportunities irrespective of race, gender, or sexual orientation. Confronted by a new colleague who claimed that this commitment was merely a reflection of their preferences – and that he or she happened to have different preferences – they would most probably be appalled. And if these health promoters went on to assert, as they well might, that their new colleague was 'in the wrong' they would not see this only as an expression of their preferences but as a claim that with regard to certain very important matters their new colleague was mistaken. In this context they may be happy to echo the sceptic's words about physics or history rather than those which are dismissive of ethics – 'There is some kind of underlying reality about which they are trying to make a judgement. There are better and worse answers to these questions and when they revise their views it is because they come to see a better answer, an answer that is "closer to the truth".'

It should be clear that these two popular currents are incompatible with each other. We cannot both think that (a) conflicting ethical beliefs are always 'equally valid' and that (b) conflicting ethical beliefs can, at least sometimes, be evaluated by considering their respective justifications, and some ethical answers are 'better' (more defensible) than others. It is necessary to decide which of these positions you accept. You cannot accept them both.

Appraising ethical judgements

Applied ethics is based on the acceptance of position (b). It can be seen as a disciplined and systematic effort to put it into practice, i.e. to examine and appraise the justification of ethical claims. Earlier we deliberately used the expression 'ethical assessment' to convey the idea that the ethical content of health promotion practices and policies can be analysed and assessed. We also wished to suggest that this analysis can and should go beyond description; that it must also involve the 'quality control' of ethical reasoning.

When someone makes an ethical claim about health promotion (or anything else) they are relying upon many things including: (i) a background framework of ethical beliefs; (ii) a large number of empirical judgements about the world – both general beliefs and beliefs about particular cases; and (iii) a more or less explicit practical judgement that links these ethical and empirical beliefs to the case in question. Applied ethics is concerned with evaluating the actual and potential reasons which underpin (i) and (iii). (It is not directly concerned with the evaluation of empirical claims but the content of these claims is important and effects the overall evaluation.) About any ethical belief or judgement we can ask, 'Is this just stated as a 'given' or are there some reasons offered to support it?' If there are reasons offered we can critically examine them. If not, then we should recognise that we are being asked to accept something uncritically.

Although the 'quality control' procedures of academic ethics will not offer definitive and conclusive evaluations we can expect it to produce 'better' rather than 'worse' answers. Furthermore the alternative is to revert to position (a) and accept some form of relativism – and the price of this is high! It would, for example, mean that we would have to accept our anti-racist and racist colleagues as occupying equally valid positions.

As we noted in the introduction to Section Two some philosophers have argued that ethical appraisal must, at some basic level, boil down to the evaluation and weighing of the consequences of actions. An action's rightness or wrongness must fundamentally depend upon the overall balance of beneficial or harmful consequences that flow from it. Others argue that this way of looking at things does not do justice to the full range of ethical values and motivations. In particular they argue that ethics depends upon faithful adherence to certain rules or principles which make sense on their own terms irrespective of their instrumental value. These two positions – *consequence-based* and *rule-based* conceptions of ethics – represent two of the main currents within ethical debate and hence are recurring concerns throughout this book.

If we scratch the surface we discover that each of these conceptions exists in a variety of forms and that there are numerous attempts to reconcile them, but even in the bald formulation given here we can see how they might begin to shed light on the ethics of health promotion. Health promotion is aimed at bringing about some combination of 'goods' (health, informed choice, well-being, fewer inequalities etc.). It naturally focuses upon consequences and on trying to optimise certain outcomes. But in working towards these ends health promoters run the risk of paying insufficient attention to what might be regarded as necessary ethical constraints on their actions – of intervening in people's lives (or sometimes perhaps of failing to intervene) in ways which might be judged to wrong them. Ethicists seek to theorise these things, to understand how best to think about consequences and their optimisation, how best to think about 'wrongful interference' or 'wrongful neglect', and how these concerns interact.

So what are the links between applied ethics and health promotion? We will begin by some reflections on the historical development of health care ethics and the ways in which this development is itself linked to health promotion. Then we will further specify and summarise the relevance of applied philosophy and health care ethics to health promotion.

The development of health care ethics

We take 'health care ethics' to be that part of applied ethics that critically examines the assumptions, values and arguments deployed by those working to treat illness and to restore or improve health. It is the application of ethics to health care practice and systems. (Our preferred term is 'health care ethics'. Others use terms such as 'medical ethics', or 'bioethics' for broadly the same field.)

How did health care ethics develop? The practice of applying ethics to the 'real world' of professional and occupational activity has grown enormously over the last thirty years. Within this general growth, the development of health care ethics has been particularly prominent, in fact, it could be argued that it has stimulated the growth of applied ethics in other areas. The growth can be seen through such things as the rapid rise in the number of 'health care ethics' courses at universities: the development of academic journals devoted to the subject; and the inclusion of ethics in the education and training curricula for health care professionals such as nurses and doctors (English National Board 1987, General Medical Council 1983). We are talking about these sorts of developments particularly in the UK context, but parallels can be found in most, if not all, developed countries. Indeed, the growth of health care ethics in the United States – which sometimes claims the actual 'birth' of health care ethics (Jonsen 1998) – has been even more profound. In the USA, for a number of years, many hospitals have employed professional ethicists to support the ethical decision-making of their clinical staff (Gorovitz 1990).

But why did all this happen? There are a number of linked reasons. In the first place, from about the 1960s and early 1970s, health care generally, and medicine particularly, were starting to be subjected to societal scrutiny and to objections in a way that had never previously happened. Critics, such as Ivan Illich (1977), Thomas McKeown (1976) and Ian Kennedy (1983), challenged medicine in various ways. Attacks on the assumptions, made by supporters of medicine, that it was without doubt a good thing, and that single-handedly it had made the twentieth century one of greater health and longevity than any previously, were especially prominent – and especially effective.

Secondly, and part of the reason why these attacks were so successful, was that medicine and health care were themselves rapidly developing at this time. Through technology, doctors were developing the capabilities to begin lives as well as to end them: to sustain them where previously someone would have died, or be considered to be dead; and to adapt and modify the lives that they were creating. To at least some extent, public reaction to these startling technological capabilities was one of worry and concern. When was 'starting life' or 'ending life' through medical practice justifiable? Should lives be created when it seemed that 'nature didn't intend it'? What would it mean for humanity if we could move towards the gradual elimination of imperfections in people? All of these questions highlighted the social and professional power of doctors. And, as we have indicated elsewhere, professional power in general was under growing public scrutiny with increasing calls for checks and balances from both managers and 'consumers' of health care. The emerging criticisms of medicine and the public worry about the technological directions it was taking were key in stimulating the rise of health care ethics. Furthermore the rising costs of health care – for a variety of reasons – focussed attention upon the control and management of health care resources, including financial, physical and 'human' resources.

Critique, loss of public confidence, and resource constraints, are some of the reasons for the rise of health care ethics during the last part of the twentieth century. But all of these factors – and in particular the critique of biomedicine – were also influential in the rise of the health promotion movement. The 1974 Lalonde Report, 'A New Perspective on the Health of Canadians' (Lalonde 1974), for example, which some regard as the first emergence of the idea of health promotion, suggested that hospital medical services by themselves could not raise the health status of a population, that broader conceptions of the nature of health were needed, and that other less professionally dominated models of health improvement were required. There is, in many respects, a broad match between the circumstances surrounding the birth of health care ethics on the one hand, and of health promotion on the other.

Some might argue, in the case of health promotion, that what was 'born' was a completely new way of understanding health and ways of creating 'more health'. We would agree that the rhetoric and the energy surrounding health promotion have the appearance of novelty in the time and the literature following Lalonde and the various early WHO charters relating to health promotion, but we doubt that in substance 'health promotion' contained much that had not happened before. The idea of 'healthy public policy' (public policy being made to work for the good of health), for example, can be identified much earlier in accounts of British social history: from Victorian public health reforms, through the earliest signs of social insurance at the beginning of the twentieth century to food policy during the second world war, and the actual creation, post-war, of the welfare state. So while the 1970s might have spawned a novel term, 'health promotion', it is by no means clear that many new practices emerged. (We are not suggesting that new ways of describing – and by implication, thinking about – things are not in themselves important. They clearly can be.)

Similarly, we would argue that when health care ethics was 'born', in many ways it was not doing things that were very much different from what some philosophers had been doing long before the end of the twentieth century. This may seem an odd claim, given that health care ethicists often apply themselves to thinking about constantly changing health care organisations, practices and technology in policy-relevant contexts. However, the ways in which this work is done typically relies heavily on lengthy traditions of ethical thinking. For example, it draws heavily on the two major traditions of theorising ethical obligations that we already discussed: consequentialism or consequence-based ethics; and deontology or rule-based ethics. If you look at how a number of key health care ethicists themselves describe their purpose, you will see them talking about the need for frameworks to restore conceptions of the ethical obligations of health care workers, challenged by recent technological and social developments (Beauchamp & Childress 1994): the requirement for principles to tell us if (and if yes, when) we have an ethical obligation to save life (Glover 1977); and the need for health care ethics to be able to support particular lines of action or conduct in individual cases (Gillon 1990). All this frequently leads health care ethicists to theories of ethical obligation, and a discussion of how to manage the tensions between rival theories and how to apply them to practice.

It is not surprising that applied philosophers, responding to the critiques of medicine and the new challenges of health care, have drawn on the long traditions of ethical thinking with which they were familiar. But the fact that philosophers turned to these areas of practical inquiry at all was itself very significant, because for much of the twentieth century, many philosophers had become preoccupied with very narrow, technical questions; and they had largely abandoned the belief that philosophy had important things to say about how humans should conduct themselves. Health care ethics – and the applied philosophy movement of which it is an important part – has restored philosophy to a crucial position in the middle of our practical lives. It has brought the theoretical and critical resources of a disciplined approach to ethical thinking into the service of health professionals and others. This presence is, of course, not always a welcome one, because applied ethicists are as capable of condemning, as of defending, the standards of professional ethics. In the remainder of the chapter, however, we will present this role in a constructive light.

Applying health care ethics to health promotion

How can health care ethics help us to understand and evaluate health promotion? From the direction of this book, it should be clear that we can seek support from health care ethics for at least three things:

- Clarifying and debating concepts and values
- Clarifying and debating the ethical acceptability of policies and practices
- Clarifying and debating what it means to be a 'good' practitioner

Clarifying and debating concepts and values

Arguably the core function of applied philosophy is to critically examine the 'frameworks of thought' with which we operate. Whether we are working within academic disciplines, social organisations or practical activities we are necessarily relying upon partly explicit and partly implicit frameworks of thinking. Applied philosophers are interested in uncovering and clarifying these frameworks, and assessing their strengths and weaknesses. A large part of this task involves focussing on the key concepts in a framework and analysing the various meanings of these concepts. To some this can seem a rather dry and academic exercise. But to anyone with a feel for applied philosophy, this process of conceptual exploration is not merely an interesting exercise but an exercise of immense 'real world' importance.

Hopefully we have given a little illustration of this practical importance in relation to the concept of health. Given that there are multiple, and often competing, accounts of what is meant by 'health', there will be analogous disputes about the purposes (and in turn, therefore, the processes) of health promotion. But we have not even begun to do justice to the potential insights and difficulties flowing from an in-depth analysis of 'health' and health-related concepts. Philosophical work on alternative conceptions of health and their implications (e.g. Nordenfelt 1993a) raises fundamental questions about the competing frameworks through which we seek to understand ourselves as human beings. Is it possible to give an objective and neutral classification of disease states (and their demarcation from non-disease states), and if so, can this provide us with a neutral and definitive account of health and its management? More generally, how far can and should we see ourselves – and what matters in our lives – through the lens of biology or any other scientific framework? And if and where that proves inadequate what other 'lenses' are available? In other words the conceptual exploration of concepts such as 'disease', 'disability', 'illness', 'ill-health', 'quality of life', 'well-being' and so on, is intimately bound up with a whole range of far reaching philosophical and practical concerns.

There are, of course, many other concepts closely linked to the field of health promotion, all of which can be subject to philosophical analysis. What do health promoters (or others) mean when they talk about, for example, responsibility, empowerment, or inequality? We have tried to give some indication of the ambiguities and contests surrounding key terms such as these, but we have not debated them at any length. It is possible to find an extensive ongoing discussion of the whole range of social concepts in the philosophical literature, but we should also stress that applied philosophy is not simply about 'seeing what is in the books' – it is a practical activity with which individuals need to engage personally. Each of us would benefit from analysing the concepts that we rely on – what exactly do I mean by 'this' or 'that'? What are the other possibilities? What are the assumptions and justifications underpinning my own use, and what are the implications for other people? If, let us say, I am a passionate advocate of community development work, have I really thought through the problems of understanding the concept 'community'? Am I, for instance, confident that I am not simply imposing the wishes of an arbitrarily circumscribed group upon others?

One important characteristic of all the concepts we have discussed is that they have an 'evaluative' as well as a 'descriptive' function. For example, when health promoters draw attention to 'inequalities' in health they are not usually merely labelling something in the way that you might label a taxi or a telephone kiosk. Of course there is, in this case, a descriptive job being done – roughly speaking it is being said that one group of people are systematically exposed to worse health experiences than another, in some respects, comparable group. But, more often than not, implicit in this use of the idea of inequalities is a value judgement of some sort. Typically what is being said (or implied) is that this difference in health experience is somehow unfair or wrong; and often linked to this, that steps ought to be taken to try to reduce this unfairness. Thus clarifying and exploring the use of concepts such as these is also clarifying and exploring value judgements. As we have noted throughout, 'health' itself has both descriptive and evaluative functions – health is a value. In passing, we have discussed a number of other key values (such as those associated with the four principles approach – autonomy, benefit, harm and justice) and all of these really require more sustained analysis and reflection than we have been able to offer. A number of health care ethicists have explored health promotion values in their writings (Campbell 1976, 1990, Cribb 1993, Cribb & Dines 1993, Dougherty 1993, Nordenfelt 1993b, Seedhouse 1997, Yeo 1993). Michael Yeo, for example, argues that for individuals and communities to be properly seen as 'healthy', they must also be free or autonomous; 'health' without freedom is not true health at all. So – for him as for many others – autonomy occupies a central place in the set of values connected to health promotion. Downie *et al.* (1996) list a set of what they call 'necessary personal values' and 'necessary social values'. These include the values of physical integrity and health, justice and the capacity to be self-determining. We will not attempt to analyse, or discuss the relationships between these sorts of values here, but perhaps some brief general reflections on values are worth offering.

To say something is a value is simply to say that it is characteristically treated as a valuable thing. Almost anything could be valuable to someone from time to time, or in specific sets of circumstances, but certain things are commonly treated as valuable almost irrespective of circumstances. Both health and autonomy are plausible candidates for this position. Furthermore, certain value concepts have the idea of 'being valuable' built into them (e.g. 'well-being', 'benefit') and the issue is deciding upon the range of application of these terms. Things can be valuable because they are necessary means to a valuable end, or they can, like well-being, be valuable as ends. Of course many things can be valuable in both senses – education is both instrumentally and intrinsically valuable. There is, then, a multitude of interesting questions about values which we will not pursue here. (For example, are some sorts of things valuable always and everywhere? Is value a product of things being treated as valuable by people, or is it rather that people recognise the value in things?) All we want to do is briefly summarise three of the main issues that quickly come to the surface when discussing values – issues that are the 'bread and butter' of work in applied ethics.

First, as we have stressed so far, the meaning of value terms is subject to ambiguity and debate. We should never assume that just because two people are using the same word (autonomy, justice etc.) that they are talking about the same thing. Second (assuming we have achieved some agreement about the meaning of certain values), the world is such that it is not possible to have all valuable things at once. There have to be trade-offs of various kinds between values. Some of the time, for example, promoting health and promoting autonomy will be compatible ends, and sometimes they will be conflicting ones, and in the latter case one or the other will have to take priority. Third, the weighing and balancing of 'packages of values' will vary between people and groups. Not only values but also judgements about priority relations between them are contestable. This, therefore, gives rise to a whole 'second level' of value judgements – judgements about what are the right principles and procedures for managing this value pluralism.

Clarifying and debating the ethical acceptability of policies and practices

What is it ethically acceptable for a health promoter to do? This is the main question lying behind the discussions in Section Two of the book. Is it always ethically acceptable for a health promoter to counsel a clinically obese client to change their lifestyle? Ought a health promoter to work on a programme which makes emergency contraception more accessible to 14 year old girls? And so on. For the most part we have discussed these kinds of questions with a view to encouraging a more ethically aware and analytical reflective practice. We have not, for the most part, argued for particular answers to these questions – although in a number of places the line of our discussion will have pointed in some directions more than in others. This emphasis upon 'opening up' rather than on 'answering' ethical questions is in keeping with our aims for this book. But outside of these aims there are other reasons to hesitate before offering answers – reasons which we will rehearse in a moment. But first we should stress that merely 'opening up' questions is not sufficient either for an applied philosopher or for a practitioner. As we have noted the applied philosopher takes seriously the task of sifting better answers from worse ones; and practitioners are in any case *forced* to 'answer' these questions (more or less reflectively) through their choices and actions.

Why hesitate to answer questions about what we ought to do? Because (a) the answers we give depend upon the frameworks of ethical thinking we deploy, and these are themselves contestable; (b) it is often difficult to generalise about answers because they depend so much on a case-by-case consideration; (c) whether generalising or considering a specific context, making ethical judgements depends upon making empirical judgements, and the latter are frequently uncertain or controversial. We will say a little more about each of these points.

To talk about 'frameworks of ethical thinking' is not the same as to talk about ethical theory because people's thinking does not necessarily correspond with the structures and forms of rationality of theoretical ethics. Nonetheless ethical theory provides a rich set of resources for exploring not only how we might happen to think but also how we *ought* to think. In the discussion (earlier in this chapter) about appraising ethical judgement we briefly illustrated the contrasting implications of consequence-based and rule-based thinking for health promotion. Roughly speaking for the former the ethical acceptability of health promotion policies and practices depends on whether they 'provide the goods', and for the latter judgements of acceptability place weight upon certain kinds of actions being ethically 'required' or 'ruled out' largely independently of their consequences. (We also noted that this is a rather broad-brush distinction and that in applied philosophy these positions are both qualified and combined in complex ways.) Even this crude distinction between different sorts of emphasis in ethical thinking helps to illuminate the challenge of ethically appraising health promotion interventions.

Take the following two very general kinds of questions (which we have met before in various guises): If certain interventions are likely to substantially improve the health experience of the population but involve an element of compulsion – when and how far is that ethically acceptable? If the same interventions involve forcing a few people to do (or experience) things that they positively do not want to do, or regard as wrong, or which causes some other harm to them – when and how far is that ethically acceptable? It should be obvious that the kinds of responses we are inclined to make to these kinds of questions will depend upon *what we think ethics is* – that is to say on the frameworks of ethical thinking we use. Any serious applied ethics must, therefore, include the articulation and defence of the grounds and the theoretical frameworks of ethics. Shorthand formulae like the four principles approach are a useful starting point for many but only a starting point. It is easy to imagine other accounts of ethical thinking. It could be argued, say, that the most important thing a health care worker could do would be to protect his or her patient or client. If so paternalism would become the pre-eminent ethical obligation. There are different views on the nature of human dignity, responsibility and freedom (Englehardt Jr & Wildes 1994), which lead to different perceptions of the obligations we ought to accept. Hence there is no easy closure on debates in health care ethics. If we wish to defend some health promotion practice we need also to be able to defend the framework of ethical thinking that underpins our position. For that we will have to turn to ethical theory.

The two general questions set out above to make a point about the contested nature of ethical thinking (and many other questions like them) are also, obviously, of great substantive significance. Different answers to them will generate very different regimes of health promotion work. Some people will argue that population health gains (or other, sometimes contrasting, public health goals such as reducing inequalities) can often justify the overriding of some wants, interests or other values. Other people will stress the importance of respecting the interests and preferences even of small numbers of individuals, and doing so even if this thwarts substantial health promotion goals. The arguments offered in support of these contrasting positions will inevitably draw upon debates in political philosophy as well as in social ethics. As we mentioned in Chapter Two there are longstanding debates in political philosophy about the legitimacy of the state, or of professional groups, intervening in individuals' lives for the sake of some conception of the public good. Ethical arguments about health promotion are always likely to be framed, in part, by these same debates. From the standpoint of occupational or professional ethics it is important to have some insight into these general debates, but they are only part of the story. They may push in a more or less interventionist position, but they rarely resolve questions about the acceptability of particular interventions. This is because every individual case is different. In reality every case involves weighing up the balance between significantly different 'packages of values', and doing so in indefinitely variable sets of circumstances. Even superficially equivalent interventions can start to look very different when they are examined under an ethical 'microscope'. (Try, for example, comparing the case for the enforcement of car seat-belt use and bicycle helmet use.) But many potential health promotion interventions are obviously very different in their value 'costs' and 'benefits'. And an intervention that is defensible in one set of circumstances may not be so in other circumstances. Health care ethicists are very used to working with this challenge and their methods and arguments have relevance to all practitioners. For example, health promoters should systematically ask themselves whether they are being *consistent* in the ethical appraisal of policies and practices. If they regard one intervention as ethically acceptable but another seemingly similar intervention as unacceptable they should discipline themselves to specify the *relevant differences* between the two cases. This will force them to be rigorous in their own thinking, and prepare them to explain their reasoning to others.

As we have discussed in various places in this book a substantial part of the difficulty of making definitive ethical appraisals, and in making these appraisals publicly defensible, is that ethical judgements are interwoven with empirical judgements. These latter might be relatively specific or they can be very general. We will simply mention one example of each kind: What is the evidence that bicycle helmet use prevents significant morbidity, and how does its preventive potential compare to that which might be derived from a substantial increase in cycle lanes? What evidence do we have to believe that it is possible for governments to use re-distributive taxation in a way that contributes both to overall economic efficiency and to greater fairness? We will not discuss these kinds of questions here because they are not in themselves questions in applied or health care ethics. However it is clear that both the relatively focused and the more general sort of empirical questions pose substantial methodological and philosophical difficulties. They are very difficult to answer indeed. Yet, as we have said, judging the ethical acceptability of health promotion depends upon answering them or, at least, on taking up a view on how to handle the uncertainty associated with them.

There are, therefore, reasons to hesitate before arguing for or against the ethical acceptability of health promotion policies and practices. But the only alternative to 'throwing up our hands' and simply ducking the issues is systematic and sustained engagement with them. We should look for the best ethical appraisals of interventions available whilst paying full regard to the difficulties of so doing. This is at the heart of the potential contribution of applied philosophy and health care ethics to health promotion.

Clarifying and debating what it means to be a 'good' practitioner

What do we mean when we talk about 'being a good practitioner'? In a general sense, this might mean someone who was good at promoting health. In other words that he or she was skilled at identifying need; at planning and implementing health promotion action aimed at meeting that need; that these actions were successful; and that the practitioner was able to evaluate this success. But in this book we have focussed upon and worked around the notion of professional ethics. We have envisaged a practitioner who is trying to do a good job, but who is also thereby interested in thinking about values and ethics. In the process we have indirectly attributed a number of qualities to this hypothetical practitioner – we have portrayed him or her as questioning, as reflective, as analytical. We have also argued, for example, that if his or her practice is to be seen as 'good practice' he or she must be *willing* to consult with their clients and to explain the reasons for their actions. In other words whilst we have concentrated upon questions about the evaluation of health promoters' actions we have also said a few things about the evaluation of health promoters themselves. What are the personal and professional qualities needed to be an ethically good health promoter? This is also an area where applied philosophy and health care ethics has a lot of relevance to offer; and although it is not something that we have chosen to review at length we feel it is worth at least introducing the relevance of this work.

Health care ethics – as an academic activity – faces analogous difficulties to codes of ethics. In some respects it falls short of helping people 'know how' to apply ethical judgements, or more generally to 'think ethically'. In the end these things require practical knowledge as well as theoretical knowledge, and in turn this rests upon the practitioners having the right sorts of commitments, motivations and orientation to their work. It is impossible to develop the skills of practical ethical thinking without a genuine personal concern and involvement with ethics (in this respect ethics is no different from any other skilled activity). So ethical theory cannot, by itself, deliver ethical practice but it can help to illuminate its nature.

Ethical theory can make a contribution to the ethical appraisal of people's characters and in particular to what might be called 'practical expertise' in ethics. Many recent philosophers, including many working within health care ethics, have turned to the Aristotelian tradition of ethics (and some more recent variants of it) to illuminate the importance of practical knowledge and the qualities of character (the virtues) which, so to speak, 'deliver' ethics. Aristotle's ethics (Aristotle 1955) shows that whilst the *identification* of virtues such as courage and justice is important, what is really essential to practical ethics is the *cultivation* of the virtues through good practice. The modern philosophical debates about this centre on 'virtue theory' (e.g. Slote 1983), which is often presented as the third major tradition in ethical theorising (making a threefold distinction between consequence-based, rule-based and character-based theory). The name of 'virtues' is given to those relatively stable and admirable dispositions of character, which provide the vehicle for ethical action. Without these qualities the abstract intellectual appraisal of policies and practices would be virtually irrelevant because there would be no reason to suppose that health promoters would act in the way these appraisals suggest. Health care ethicists have now done a substantial amount of work on character and health care professionals, and this work has as much relevance to health promotion as to other kinds of health work. We will say more about the idea of the virtues and their role in health promotion in the next chapter under the heading of 'personal integrity'. But before concluding this chapter we want to add a few notes about another aspect of the Aristotelian perspective on the ethical judgement of people's lives.

For virtue theorists the cultivation of an individual's character serves two closely married purposes – it helps to support and facilitate desirable and worthwhile communities (as we have said virtues are the vehicle of ethical action), and it realises the possibility of a worthwhile life for the individual concerned. Virtues support the living of 'good lives' both socially and personally. This notion of investigating what it is to live a worthwhile or good life is an enormously important one in applied ethics and is at least as old as Socrates (Haldane 1986). It is an aspect of ethics which is sometimes neglected in contemporary discussions, perhaps because it is seen as rather archaic or judgmental by some people (although the same people may be happy to ask this question about their own lives). But it is certainly not a question that can be ignored by health promoters, because amongst their number are many who see their work as about promoting well-being. Indeed everyone who works in health promotion must have regard to the fact that some health promoters think in these terms. This means that health promoters are themselves often thinking about what it means for people to live worthwhile or good lives, and of ways of helping to support this. To this extent there is a real overlap between the Aristotelian tradition and the 'frameworks of thinking' of some health promotion. 'Well-being promoters' are not simply interested in how to minimise the disease experience of populations, rather they want to see their work as about helping people to live full and fulfilling lives; and in turn this requires them to think through what actually is meant by ideas like this. Virtue theory has the potential to be a substantial help in this task. Ethical analysis in this area can support both a constructive and sceptical function. On the one hand it can help health promoters find models and concepts which allow them to articulate and debate ideas around well-being, fulfilment and so on. On the other hand it can point up the danger of health promoters uncritically importing their own personal conceptions of 'good lives' – or conceptions deriving from professional norms or government norms about the public good – into their work. Whatever else it is to be a good health promotion practitioner it surely does not involve judging other lives through one's own prejudices.

Conclusion

In this chapter, we have discussed a number of ways in which health care ethics is able to help those engaged with the practical difficulties of promoting health. We have suggested that health care ethics is particularly useful in clarifying and debating the values and assumptions embodied in health promotion policy and practice, and the ethical acceptability of health promotion policies and practices. And we have noted that both of these things are necessary – but not sufficient – for the ethical development of good health promotion practitioners. Health promoters also need to develop an ethical orientation through a serious personal involvement in 'ethical thinking' – a personal involvement and thinking which is practically oriented. This includes the inclinations, feelings and skills which support day-to-day ethical judgement – the cultivation of virtues. But it also involves an accompanying readiness to reflect on fundamental questions about the nature of the good life, and in particular on the role of health promotion in building worthwhile and meaningful human lives.

Chapter 9
Some Resources for the
Reflective Health Promoter

Introduction

We have tended for the most part in this book to emphasise the open-ended, contested and complex nature of health promotion values and ethics. In doing so, our aim has been to subvert the superficially plausible – but highly dangerous – assumption that health promotion is simply and only 'a good thing'. However there are also dangers associated with such subversion. In bringing to the foreground the mass of complexities and ethical ambiguities facing health promoters, we have risked undermining their capacity and confidence to 'get on with the job'. Given all the uncertainties we have drawn out, an individual health promoter might say – 'I don't know where to begin!'

In passing we should note that this reaction is not necessarily a bad one; arguably, it is preferable to a dogmatic insistence on the merits of one's activities. In this final chapter, though, we hope to shift the emphasis a little. Ultimately, our goal in writing this book is to support the work of health promoters. This has been our goal throughout the discussion and debate in which we have engaged. Our belief is that the critical reflection we hope we have encouraged is vital to 'good practice' in health promotion. Our aim now, in this chapter, is to draw together some of the threads of our book: to focus on the resources available to support reflective health promotion; and so actively to move towards use in practice of the debates we have had and the thinking we hope to have encouraged. The term 'resources' is being used here in its most general sense: if health promoters are looking for support with ethical issues, where should they look; what should they be looking for; and who might be able to help them? We will shortly set out a range of appropriate 'starting points' for addressing these questions. First, however, we will set the scene by discussing the nature of the relationship between ethics and 'the reflective health promoter'.

Customary and reflective ethics

A number of writers and academics have made a distinction between two different dimensions of ethics. On the one hand there is the ethics of custom, habit or convention – the 'taken for granted' ethics of day-to-day practice. On the other hand there is the critical ethics of analytic philosophy – that aspect of ethics which 'stands back from' day-to-day ethics and analyses it, challenges it or seeks to improve on it. We can call the first dimension of ethics customary ethics; and the second dimension reflective ethics. This distinction between customary and reflective ethics has links with (but is not the same as) that which we have just been making between 'constructive' and 'subversive' perspectives on ethics. However, we wish to stress that both customary and reflective ethics – in combination – have a practical and constructive role. They are both required. And for health promoters, there is a need to identify resources to support both dimensions.

If we think about our day-to-day lives, it is possible to begin seeing why both customary and reflective ethics are necessary. Family life, and our wider social lives, depend upon multi-layered patterns of social co-operation. Among these patterns are more or less explicit rules of conduct, norms and mutual expectations. Together, these patterns produce a 'climate of ethics and values' which penetrates our whole lives. We know how we should drive our cars, walk down the street, queue for tickets, hold a conversation at work or amongst friends, eat our food and so on. As an important part of such 'knowledge', we can identify many things we should not do: some of which are seen as 'eccentric' or 'bad manners'; and some of which are 'wrong'. If I am invited round to a friend for dinner, I might take along a bottle of wine. It would be bad form to turn up very late, especially without apologising even if I was clutching my bottle of wine. It would be eccentric and rather bad manners of me to expect to be given my bottle back if it had not been drunk during the meal. And it would be plain wrong if I were to use the opportunity to help myself to my friend's prized possessions! We 'know' that stealing is wrong. In fact, we are probably talking not so much of 'knowledge' that stealing is wrong, as of a firm and quite likely entrenched belief. Under normal circumstances we do not feel that it is necessary to analyse or 'challenge' this belief. What is more we are likely to be suspicious of any attempt to undertake such a process of challenge. We are wary about undermining norms which hold our social fabric together.

It is easy to see why customary ethics is needed. It enables our social lives and relationships to continue in ways that are generally acceptable to most people for most of the time. However, a few moments' thought also demonstrates the necessity for reflective ethics. What are we to say to those people who say they 'know' that homosexuality or inter-racial marriages are wrong? We can easily imagine they have the same kind of conviction about these things as we do about stealing. Let us also imagine they come from a culture or sub-culture in which their views are the norm; and where the general view is that the 'practices' they condemn, if allowed, would certainly undermine the social fabric of their society. Clearly we cannot say that these views are ethically acceptable simply because they reflect custom and practice. Customary ethics is necessary for our daily lives but it is not sufficient to justify particular positions we might hold. Nothing can be accepted simply on the basis that it is customary. We have to be able to critically reflect on, and challenge, customary ethics. We need to look for good reasons either to support or to revise the claims of customary ethics. (This echoes the argument we made at the beginning of Chapter 8 in support of academic ethics.)

As it is the case in every day life, the task for health promoters is to combine, and find the right balance between customary and reflective ethics. They need to establish customary norms and expectations to facilitate their work and relationships. They also need, though, to be reflective about – and critical of – these customary norms and expectations. Too much focus on custom at the expense of reflection risks building unacceptable values into the fabric of their work. And too much focus on reflection at the expense of custom can engender inactivity and a sense of being without any kind of normative beliefs whatsoever. (It is important to have a neutral gear in a car, but you will never go anywhere in neutral.) The previous two chapters have each emphasised one of these two dimensions of customary and reflective ethics. On the one hand, the project of developing, disseminating and making reference to 'codes of ethics' is an influential aspect of the dimension of customary ethics. It helps to articulate mutual expectations and shared norms. (It is no coincidence that codes of ethics are mostly generated and driven by members of the occupation or profession concerned.) On the other hand, the contribution of applied philosophy to ethics is principally about critical appraisal and analysis – it is the most influential medium of reflective ethics.

As we tried to illustrate in earlier chapters (particularly Chapters 1 and 2), one of the difficulties facing health promoters is that there is little by way of a specific 'customary ethic' in health promotion. Those health promoters who occupy 'traditional' health professional roles (for example, as nurses or doctors) do have recourse to a whole array of resources. These include: evolving but well known models of professional-client relationships; long established codes and guidelines; professional bodies who monitor or oversee practice and so on. We will return to some of these kinds of resources shortly. It is important at this point, though, to note that in a number of important respects, the adoption of a health promotion function disrupts such resources and potentially threatens their relevance. At the very least, it requires that clients entering into a relationship with health professionals who have adopted this function understand that the professionals' focus and priorities may have shifted somewhat. For example, a primary health care patient being offered a vaccination or screening needs to have made explicit to him or her – if we are being serious about the idea of 'informed consent' in health promotion – that the professional's motivation may be as much population health as her or his own individual well-being.

By contrast, health promotion specialists are much less likely to face such specific forms of role ambiguity and expectation (as represented by the example here, the tension between individual-responsive and population-promotion roles). They do not have to worry about whether their customary ethic will 'stretch' adequately. As we have noted, though, they face an even bigger problem – the relative lack of a rich customary ethic at all. (Apart, that is, from the general societal ethics in which they work – which is, of course, an important common resource.) While some practitioners have wrestled with the development of a code of ethics for specialist health promotion, as we discussed in Chapter 7: and while an increasing number of theorists have applied themselves to the demands of an ethics for health promotion; none of this really adds up to a specific 'customary ethic' for the field. This latter would entail that there is a 'living', taken for granted, framework of values and ethics understood and accepted at least by health promotion specialists, but ideally by both the specialists and the populations of clients their work affects. We suggest there is perhaps the beginnings of such a shared understanding amongst some groups of health promotion specialists but it would be very difficult to argue there is anything much more than a beginning.

This should not be taken as a criticism of the field of health promotion. It is largely a consequence of the fact that the field is relatively new. One of the shortcomings of a reliance on customary ethics – implied but not spelled out above – is that such ethics take time to coalesce around a set of practices. They are therefore likely to have 'little to say about' emerging fields and activities. It is also a product of the fact that much health promotion work takes place 'at a distance' between practitioners and clients and these more distant relationships fall outside our traditional ethical perceptions and vocabularies. Under these circumstances there is an especially important role for a reflective approach to ethics. Health promotion involves new customs and practices. It therefore requires a 'new' professional ethics. It will be clear now why it is particularly important to assemble and marshal all of the resources which can help support and develop a professional ethics for health promoters – resources for both customary and reflective ethics.

We suggest that health promoters need to draw together a number of complementary approaches and perspectives – *visions, health promotion theory, applied ethics, professional traditions, standards of good practice* and *personal integrity*. They need to draw these things together in a way that combines a personal capacity for critical reflexivity with the formation of an ethical 'community of practice' (Lave & Wenger 1991). In what follows we will develop these thoughts further. We will summarise these approaches and perspectives, but we will also explore their inter-relationships.

Health promotion visions

Health promoters are their own best resource. Whether they are promoting health from the traditional roles of health care or from the 'new' role of health promotion specialist, they typically do not think of their work as 'just a job'. Most of them will enter the field inspired by the opportunity to benefit other people and the communities in which they work. Although this idealism tends to be gradually eroded by the normal pressures and difficulties attached to any kind of employment, it will normally remain as part of their core identity. The absurdities of managing budgets and adhering to performance targets, or the petty rivalries around status and salaries, may dent their 'vocation'; but in their saner moments they can still draw on their visions and ideals for inspiration.

We will shortly enter some cautions about personal visions and ideals, and stress the need for them to be moderated by other elements. Before this, however, we wish to acknowledge their importance. Health promoters should ask themselves, and one another, questions about what motivated them to enter the field. What really matters to them about their role? What do they value about their work? What counts to them personally – not to their employers – as success? Clearly there will be a range of different answers to these questions. But a number of things are likely to feature frequently: a desire to respond to those in need or at risk; a desire to help individuals to choose better and more fulfilling lives; a desire to help address some of the inequities people face; a desire to help create a pleasanter and more hospitable environment.

These desires and the motivations underpinning them are surely admirable. It is important to note, of course, that just because an action is motivated by an admirable desire does not mean it will necessarily be 'for the good'. Good motives are not enough. But they are an important start. They provide the engine driving us towards defensible health promotion. We would argue that the visions informing health promotion are not rehearsed and celebrated as they should be. This is particularly the case in the every day work place. They are largely unspoken and taken for granted. It is as if they are rather too personal and idealistic to be admitted into the sober setting of ordinary working life.

Theories of health promotion

The reason that personal visions need to be acknowledged and spoken about is not just to celebrate them but to make them explicit – to make them accessible to colleagues and potential clients. Health promoters are accountable to their clients, the populations they serve, and to their employers and colleagues. In order to exercise this accountability, they have to be ready and willing to 'give an account' of what they are doing, of what they are about. Throughout this book, we have emphasised that health promoters are engaged in 'interfering' in the lives of others. They owe it to these others to be articulate and to defend the purpose and rationale of their work. This, we would suggest, is one of the main roles of health promotion theory – to help practitioners and their managers formulate accounts of their work.

Of course, there are other functions for theory. Epidemiology, for instance, helps health promoters to identify the places where their effort might be focused. Some social and psychological theory can, for instance, help to describe and measure the mechanisms by which interventions may or may not be effective. And there are many such ways in which theory can contribute to the technical strength of health promoters. However, technical knowledge is only really of value if we have a philosophy underpinning our work, and a philosophy which we are prepared to submit to public scrutiny and debate. This task of articulating the nature of, and justifications for, health promotion is fundamental.

Fortunately, health promotion theorists have not neglected these issues. In fact some people may feel that as a relatively new domain, it has been overly pre-occupied with them at the expense of other potential sorts of theory. There are countless articles setting out, analysing and debating models and approaches to health promotion. (See, for just a few examples of these, Beattie 1991, Downie *et al.* 1996, Ewles & Simnett 1995; Tones 1983, 1990.) Although these do not pro-vide any definitive or consensual conclusions, they do provide a rich range of vocabularies and perspectives to help health promoters in 'capturing' their role in words. Taken together, the literature of health promotion 'models' provides a rich taxonomy of the potential objectives and methods of the field. Health pro-moters should be able to articulate the different conceptions of health promotion aims and their links to the valuation of different approaches and models of evaluation. They should have a reflective awareness of the different faces of what we have called (in Section One) both 'hard' and 'soft' health promotion work. Given this, and the need for accountability, there is no justification for any inability on the part of health promoters to describe the 'ends' and the 'means' of their work. However, the ability to describe is only one side of the coin of accountability. The other essential ability is to be prepared to justify or defend. So there is an essential requirement for health promoters to engage with applied ethics.

Applied ethics

There is, perhaps, a danger of health promoters thinking that 'vision' plus theoretical models is sufficient to guide their practice. They may imagine that the models provide the language to describe and plan practice; while the vision is what legitimates this practice. But if such assumptions are made, they may pose substantial dangers to the credibility and ethical acceptability of health promo-tion. Considering an analogy with religious evangelists might make the risks clear. They too are likely to be equipped with a supporting language and vision. They are confident that they are working for the good. But it surely does not follow from these things that their efforts are necessarily ethically acceptable. We would need to examine their practices case by case and evaluate them ethically before making any such judgement. So there is a need to complement, and extend, health promotion theory to draw it towards the field of applied ethics (and *vice versa*). In fact, this is increasingly happening, with the gradual development and convergence of studies in health promotion and health care ethics.

We argued in Chapter 8 that applied ethics offers assistance to health promoters in two main ways. First, it can help with mapping and clarifying the concepts, assumptions and arguments which inform policy and practice. Second, it can assist in appraising the ethical defensibility of health promotion interventions. Of course, there will be a limit to the extent that ethical analysis is likely to produce clear and uncontested conclusions. Indeed, it is likely that the more we expose rival assumptions and competing values, the more complex the debates will become. However, this strengthens the case for applied ethics rather than weakening it; if the issues really are complex and contestable, then there is nothing admirable or 'professional' about pretending they are not.

Moreover, the process of clarifying and debating these ethical issues has in itself an intrinsic importance. First, it once again helps to spread necessary vocabularies (of ethics and values) for scrutiny and accountability. Second, and crucially, it assists in building thoughtful and critical 'communities of practice'. The use of applied ethics is relatively limited if it is simply an academic exercise undertaken in isolation by reflective individuals. However, once these reflections and debates form a part of conversation amongst colleagues, and are enacted and re-enacted as part of the routine of a professional life, they have the potential to change things considerably.

In Chapter 8 we were only able to suggest a little of the potential for an applied ethics of health promotion. But we hope that we have provided some resources for those health promoters who wish to take these issues further. In particular we hope that the network of concerns and questions that we have set out provides a useful springboard. We have tried to illustrate the ways in which health promotion interventions are closely bound up with many other social and policy processes, such that it is impossible to debate the ethics of intervention in isolation from these wider questions. This gives rise to the three 'levels' of issues we have discussed in places – ethics in the substantive fields implicated in health promotion (e.g. about sexuality); the ethical acceptability of health promotion intervention; and professional conduct and styles of working in practice. We have tried to indicate the multiple ways in which health promotion gives rise to conflicts of interests – conflicts of *benefits*, *wants* and of *values*. And we have explained and explored what we take to be four core concerns for an ethics of health promotion: empowerment or control, individuals or populations, problems of evidence and uncertainty, and legitimacy in decision-making.

Professional traditions

All health promoters are supported to some extent by professional traditions. Some practitioners will think of themselves as being 'a professional'; most are likely to aspire to do their work in a 'professional' manner. This commitment, one way or another, to 'professional' ways of working is generally deeply embedded within our culture; and particularly so within the health care sector. While, in health care, understandings of what it is to be working 'as a professional' or 'in a professional way' are evolving (and we have argued, particularly in Chapter 2, that health promotion is itself part of that evolution); nevertheless, the roots of what we might call the 'traditions of professionalism' are deep.

Those health promoters from established professions (doctors and nurses, for example) will not only have a broad cluster of practical resources to draw upon (publications, training courses, peer review and so on); they will also have a self-identity and public persona built around certain fundamental technical and ethical standards. These will include, for example, acceptance of the idea of accountability, a concern with evidence of effectiveness and models of good practice, a client-centred orientation, and the assumption that they must deal in an honest and trustworthy way with those they are trying to serve. While all professionals may slip from such standards, the point is that they form an essential part of the landscape of professionalism. Professionals do not 'opt in' to these standards – they are the default position.

Health promoters who are not part of an established profession will none-theless work in contexts, such as health care, where these standards are the norm. They will be inclined to judge their work, then, against such standards. In the case of some groups – including health promotion specialists – they will also, to some extent, develop analogous structures and practices to underpin their work. Many, understandably, will be sceptical about certain aspects of the ideology of 'the profession', for example, those which emphasise or imply the power and status of 'the professional' and the consequent exclusion from consultation and decision-making of the 'non-professional'. Even so, there are many other aspects of professional traditions that both sceptic and non-sceptic will value and want – directly or indirectly – to draw on. At the heart of these is the idea of the pro-fession as upholding and developing public 'standards of good practice'.

Standards of good practice

In Chapter 7, we discussed the value and limitations of codes of ethics in some depth. Codifying ethical standards has a role in providing both a publicly available statement and a useful set of reminders. A code cannot *make* practi-tioners ethical, but it can be a useful reference point for both educational and enforcement purposes. The same is true of other similar or related statements (for example, guidelines on aspects of professional practice): some of which cover technical standards alone; and some of which incorporate both technical and ethical aspects. The organisations representing professional groups typically produce a wide range of such documentation.

Elements of these professional frameworks have a legal standing. Sometimes they act as reminders of specific statutory duties and sometimes they provide guidance which includes consideration of relevant legal positions. It is of course essential that health promoters understand, and take into account, the law affecting their work. This is not the same as to say they must agree with it, or even necessarily abide by it. However, they will clearly need very good reasons indeed if they decide to ignore the demands of the law – to disregard it from sheer ignorance is unacceptable. Other elements of these frameworks relate more to 'professional standards' which can themselves be more or less binding within the professional group concerned.

It is not enough, however, for health promoters simply to know about the existence of standards of good practice. It is essential they are prepared to participate in debates about the role, construction, adequacy and acceptability of standards. Management of health professionals is increasingly through regulation of their 'performance'. The use of outcome and performance indicators, often detailing expectations in terms of 'acceptable practice', is increasingly prominent (Scally & Donaldson 1998). Although these performance management techniques provide a system of accountability, this system is only as valuable as the techniques employed allow. If the measures and guidelines are misjudged, or if the processes for implementing them are insensitive, then their overall impact will be negative. Health promoters may benefit from statements related to the expected outcomes of practice, but only if they are ready to be constructively critical of them. Here, debates about the models and ethics of health promotion – which may offer alternative accounts of 'effective practice' – can come into their own.

Personal integrity

Of course, personal integrity is not a resource specific to health promoters. It is an essential feature of any ethical life. Just as we value bodily integrity, so we place worth on psychological integrity – we expect our colleagues and acquaintances to exhibit a measure of consistency, coherence and stability in their attitudes and behaviour. Indeed if they did not do so we would not even be able to recognise them as the 'same person' from one time to another. (Of course, people change but not in ways that are random and constant.) Our use, though, of the expression 'personal integrity' is not intended to refer to just any kind of coherence; but rather to the existence of a coherent *ethical* life. Someone with personal integrity would be expected to have, and to act out, a relatively coherent vision of how they ought to be – a set of ethical principles and standards which they take sufficiently seriously to put into practice. Personal integrity is not about what people say; it is about who they are in practice. It is about their character.

To talk about the importance of integrity is, then, a shorthand way of referring to the range of virtues necessary to practise the ethical life – both in general, and in particular roles and circumstances. In this chapter we have already mentioned the importance of honesty and trustworthiness, and these are certainly core virtues in a professional life. We have also referred to the value of idealism under the pressure of the 'real world', the place of 'compassion' for those in need, and the motivation of 'justice' in the face of health inequalities. Other people would no doubt want to develop their own list of important virtues for health professionals including health promoters which might include some of the things we have mentioned but which would also perhaps include other kinds of virtues. There is certainly room for debate about what should be on such a list and the relative priority of the items. This, however, is not our primary concern here.

We simply wish to restate the need for what we have already called 'inside-out' ethics (Dawson 1994). Defensible health promotion (like all ethical life) requires the engine of integrity – of well motivated, conscientious and practically capable individuals. Without this, all talk of ethics is simply 'hot air'. Developing a 'vision' of your work in health promotion is certainly part of an 'inside-out' ethics. But visions need to be harnessed and moderated by virtues.

The things we have discussed – health promotion visions, theories of health promotion, applied ethics, standards of good practice, and personal integrity – are, we would suggest, some of the main resources available to support the work of health promoters. They represent a range of different kinds of starting points; different elements which may go towards a compound of ethically defensible health promotion. But how does this compound come together? What are the mechanisms for articulating the elements into a whole? In the concluding section of this chapter, and this book, we will consider these questions. In order to do so we use again the distinction we drew earlier between customary and reflective ethics. We also rely on the distinction we have used throughout this chapter – between the individual professional and the professional group.

Our position is easily stated. Indeed we hope it follows fairly clearly from our discussion so far. We will first present it in a few words and then review it in a little more depth.

> *Health promoters first need to identify their relevant 'reference group' and to identify the customary ethical resources available to that group. This provides the baseline of habits, norms and codes against which they appraise their own work. Then, individually and collectively, they need to build not only a reflective culture but also a sustained critical community that 'demands' firstly, ethical scrutiny of all health promotion work; and secondly, ethical accountability and justification of policies and practices. These processes of reflection and debate should also be used to critique, revise, or extend the prevailing customary ethics.*

Developing ethics in health promotion – a shared responsibility

Health promoters will have at least one 'reference group' – one or more group of workers with whom they can identify themselves. For some health promoters, these professional communities are clear-cut and in many instances the bonds of self-identity and group identity are quite strong. An individual may see themselves as a midwife, a GP, a health visitor, a paediatric nurse and so forth. In other cases, these fields of self and shared identity will be somewhat more diffuse and the bonds relatively weaker. A health promoter working in an environmental health department in a local authority, for example, may not have many immediate colleagues with whom they identify closely. However, they may broadly identify themselves with both environmental health specialists and health promotion specialists. We will call both these groups of workers 'professional groups' for short, but in doing so we will leave aside the contestabilities about 'professionalism' and 'professionalisation' which we have referred to in other parts of this book.

Professional groups have a crucial role in developing a defensible ethic for health promoters. Individual health promoters can and should look to their professional community for a conversation about the nature and demands of their roles, including the ethical demands and dilemmas (both implicit and explicit) they face. Over time, some of these conversations may have coalesced into codes and guidelines, but however codified the customary ethic is, these conversations are never closed. Codes need to be revised from time to time and even long established principles have to be re-interpreted and re-applied as circumstances change. This is not to say that the individual health promoter can somehow 'devolve' the responsibility for ethics to their professional group. Where ethics are concerned individuals cannot hide behind groups (we will return to this point shortly). The group, though, has some obvious advantages over the isolated individual:

(1) Ethics develops through discussion, debate and argument. Both the clarification and the justification of ethical claims requires that different perspectives are rehearsed, considered and 'tested' against one other. Dialogue within the professional community can facilitate this process.
(2) A professional group can, to a certain extent, 'make public' its shared conceptions of what is ethically required – through various authoritative publications. These public statements provide a shared reference point and shared 'ways of talking' for individual practitioners to use as a starting point in the ethical appraisal of their work.
(3) A professional group can set up formal bodies and mechanisms to 'police' individual practitioners' standards, to support and develop individuals, and to represent individuals in the event of criticism or challenges to their credibility or competence.

For all these reasons professional groups can offer influential, and often powerful, support for the individual health promoter. It would probably seem odd if someone did not think it was worth looking to their peer group for inspiration and guidance about ethics. And in practice, individuals may often feel they have no choice but to seek guidance – their livelihood and status perhaps depends on the judgements of the formal authorities within their professional community. This concentration of power in professional bodies does not mean, though, that individual practitioners are simply powerless 'subjects'.

The professional community is, in the end, only the product of the individual perceptions and efforts of its members working in various coalitions. And although professional groups can have a formal and powerful 'face' in professional associations and bodies, they can also have many other less formal faces. In seminars and workshops – or more often than not in day-to-day dialogue in the workplace – professional colleagues can share and explore ideas, criticise the *status quo*, and make recommendations for changes to their own, or local or national, priorities and standards. In short, professional communities have the potential to support critical and radical thinking as well as conformist thinking.

In other words, professional communities can support reflective ethics as well as customary ethics. As we have argued above, these two dimensions of ethics are both essential. Our prevailing habits and norms provide a taken-for-granted framework against which we understand ourselves. But we must be alive to the possibility that elements of this framework are mere convention, mere prejudice or even plain wrong. If individual health promoters are to embody and exercise personal integrity they have to be ready to question convention – applied ethics provides some tools which can help, as do debates about the models of health promotion.

All health promoters therefore, have two kinds of responsibility in relation to the development of health promotion ethics.

First, health promoters are responsible for the health promotion interventions in which they play a part – they (along with their colleagues) must be ready to explain and justify these interventions in the light of possible ethical criticism. They are directly accountable for these activities and must have an account of (a) why, on balance, they are justified; and (b) what they have done in the practical design of the intervention to maximise their ethical acceptability. But this is only one aspect of their ethical responsibility.

Second, each individual has some responsibility for developing the 'values and ethical climate' of health promotion. They have a duty to ensure that the customary ethics of their professional group is both understood and subject to reflective critique. This may seem like a rather open-ended and daunting responsibility to place on the shoulders of any individual but it is a *shared* responsibility. No one person is responsible for all of this but everyone is responsible for a part of it. In professional life it is no excuse simply to say 'I don't make the rules' – because we all have the potential and the responsibility to contribute to the ethical frameworks in which we work.

In seeking support to develop more defensible health promotion work, practitioners must look in a number of directions and to a range of other people. The clients and the populations they seek to serve have an important role in contributing to this ethical debate. First and foremost, though, health promoters must look to one another and to themselves.

References

Anderson, P., Wallace, P. & Jones, H. (1988) *Alcohol Problems*. Oxford University Press, Oxford.

Aristotle (1955) *Ethics* (translated by J.A.K. Thomson). Penguin, Harmondsworth.

Ashworth, P. (1997) Breakthrough or bandwagon? Are interventions tailored to stages of change more effective than non-staged interventions? *Health Education Journal*, **56**, 166–74.

Beattie, A. (1991) Knowledge and control in health promotion: a test case for social theory. In: *The Sociology of the Health Service* (eds J. Gabe, M. Calnan & M. Bury). Routledge, London.

Beauchamp, T.L. & Childress, J.F. (1994) *Principles of Biomedical Ethics (4th edn)*. Oxford University Press, Oxford.

Belasco, W. (1997) Food, morality and social reform. In: *Morality and Health* (eds A.M. Brandt & P. Rozin), 185–200. Routledge, New York.

Benn, P. (1999) Is sex morally special? *Journal of Applied Philosophy*, **16** (3), 235–45.

Benzeval, M., Judge, K. & Whitehead, M. (1995) *Tackling Inequalities in Health: An Agenda for Action*. King's Fund, London.

Blackburn, C. (1991) *Poverty and Health: Working with Families*. Open University Press, Milton Keynes.

Bremner, M. (1994) *Professional Development in Health Promotion: A Strategic Framework*. South Thames Regional Health Authority, London.

British Fluoridation Society (1996) *One in a Million: Water Fluoridation and Dental Public Health*. Liverpool.

Bunton, R. & Macdonald, G. (1992) *Health Promotion: Disciplines and Diversity*. Routledge, London.

Bunton, R., Nettleton, S. & Burrows, R. (1995) *The Sociology of Health Promotion: Critical Analyses of Consumption, Lifestyle and Risk*. Routledge, London.

Calnan, M. (1987) *Health and Illness: The Lay Perspective*. Tavistock, London.

Campbell, A.V. (1976) Health and human freedom. *Journal of the Institute of Health Education*, **14** (3), 67–70.

Campbell, A.V. (1990) Education or indoctrination? The issue of autonomy in health education. In: *Ethics in Health Education* (ed. S. Doxiadis), 15–28. John Wiley and Sons Ltd, Chichester.

Connolly, W. (1993) *The Terms of Political Discourse*. Blackwell, Oxford.

Cornwell, J. (1984) *Hard-Earned Lives: Accounts of Health and Illness from East London*. Tavistock, London.

Cotter, C. (1994) *Professional development of health promotion specialists: exploring diploma course provision.* MSc Thesis, South Bank University, London.

Cribb, A. (1993) The borders of health promotion: a response to Nordenfelt. *Health Care Analysis,* **1** (2), 131–7.

Cribb, A. & Dines, A. (1993) Health promotion: concepts. In: *Health Promotion Concepts and Practice* (eds A. Dines & A. Cribb), 3–64. Blackwell Scientific, Oxford.

Cribb, A. & Duncan, P. (1999) Making a profession of health promotion? Grounds for trust and health promotion ethics. *International Journal of Health Promotion and Education,* **37** (4), 129–34.

Crisp, R., Hope, T. & Ebbs, D. (1996) The Asbury draft policy on ethical use of resources. *British Medical Journal,* **312**, 1528–31.

Dawson, A.J. (1994) Professional codes of practice and ethical conduct. *Journal of Applied Philosophy,* **11** (2), 145–53.

Department of Health (1996) *NHS General Medical Services Statement of Fees and Allowances Payable to General Medical Practitioners in England and Wales.* In: *The Red Book.* Department of Health, London.

Department of Health (1998) *The New NHS: Modern, Dependable.* HMSO, London.

Department of Health (2000a) *Department of Health Guidance on Tackling Teenage Pregnancy.* Department of Health Teenage Pregnancy Unit, Department of Health, London.

Department of Health (2000b) *The NHS Plan.* Department of Health, London.

Donnelly, L. (2000) Delays in HIV funding attacked. *Health Service Journal,* 11 May, 6.

Donnison, J. (1988) *Midwives and Medical Men.* Historical Publications Ltd, London.

Dougherty, C.J. (1993) Bad faith and victim-blaming: the limits of health promotion. *Health Care Analysis,* **1**, 111–19.

Downie, R.S., Tannahill, C. & Tannahill, A. (1996) *Health Promotion: Models and Values, 2nd edn.* Oxford University Press, Oxford.

Duncan, P. (1997) *Promoting Health.* South Bank University Distance Learning Centre, London.

Duncan, P. & Cribb, A. (1996) Helping people change: an ethical approach? *Health Education Research,* **11** (3), 339–48.

Dworkin, R. (1995) *Life's Dominion: An Argument about Abortion and Euthanasia.* Harper Collins, London.

Englehardt, H.T. Jr & Wildes, K.W. (1994) The four principles of health care ethics and post-modernity: why a libertarian interpretation is unavoidable. In: *Principles of Health Care Ethics* (eds R. Gillon & A. Lloyd). John Wiley and Sons Ltd, Chichester.

English National Board for Nursing, Midwifery and Health Visiting (1987) *Managing Change in Nurse Education – Pack 1: Preparing for Change.* English National Board, London.

Enkin, M., Keirse, M.J.N.C. & Chalmers, I. (1989) *A Guide to Effective Care in Pregnancy and Childbirth.* Oxford University Press, Oxford.

European Parliament (2000) *European Policy on Food Safety: Working Document for the Directorate General for Research.* European Parliament, Luxembourg.

Ewles, L. & Simnett, I. (1995) *Promoting Health: A Practical Guide to Health Education (3rd edn).* Scutari Press, Harrow.

Family Heart Study Group (1994) Randomised controlled trial evaluating cardiovascular screening and intervention in general practice: principle results of the British family heart study. *British Medical Journal*, **308**, 313–20.

Fielding, M. (1996) Empowerment: emancipation or enervation? *Journal of Education Policy*, **11** (3), 399–417.

Fitzpatrick, M. (2001) *The Tyranny of Health: Doctors and the Regulation of Lifestyle*. Routledge, London.

Food Standards Agency (2000) *Food Standards Agency Web Site*. Food Standards Agency (www.foodstandards.gov.uk) (3 July).

General Medical Council (1993) *Tomorrow's Doctors*. General Medical Council, London.

Gillon, R. (1990) *Philosophical Medical Ethics*. John Wiley and Sons Ltd, Chichester.

Gillon, R. (1994) Medical ethics: four principles plus attention to scope. *British Medical Journal*, **309**, 184–8.

Glover, J. (1977) *Causing Death and Saving Lives*. Penguin, Harmondsworth.

Gordon, L. (1997) Teenage pregnancy and out-of-wedlock birth: morals, moralism, experts. In: *Morality and Health* (eds A.M. Brandt & P. Rozin), 251–270. Routledge, New York.

Gorovitz, S. (1985) *Doctors' Dilemmas: Moral Conflict and Medical Care*. Oxford University Press, New York.

Gorovitz, S. (1990) Health care advertising: communication or confusion? In: *Ethics in Health Education* (ed. S. Doxiadis), 45–62. John Wiley and Sons Ltd, Chichester.

Graham, H. (1993) *When Life's a Drag: Women, Smoking and Disadvantage*. HMSO, London.

Haldane, J.J. (1986) 'Medical ethics' – an alternative approach. *Journal of Medical Ethics*, **12**, 145–50.

Handy, C. (1985) *Understanding Organisations*, 3rd edn. Penguin, London.

Hare, R.M. (1986) Health. *Journal of Medical Ethics*, **12**, 174–81.

Hawe, P., Degeling, D. & Hall, J. (1990) *Evaluating Health Promotion*. Maclean and Petty Pty Ltd, Artarmon, NSW.

Health Education Authority (1993) *Helping People Change: Training Course for Primary Health Care Professionals*. Health Education Authority, London.

Health Service Journal (2000a) Ovarian cancer drug will cost health authorities millions. *Health Service Journal*, 11 May, 5.

Health Service Journal (2000b) Poll victory for A and E campaigners. *Health Service Journal*, 11 May, 8.

Health Service Journal (2000c) Ventilator trial inquiry finds significant errors. *Health Service Journal*, 11 May, 4.

Herzlich, C. (1973) *Health and Illness*. Academic Press, London.

Hird, V. (2000) *Perfectly Safe to Eat?* Women's Press Ltd, London.

Hudson, F. (1999) Sex and relationships education in the secondary school. In: *Evidence-Based Health Promotion* (eds E. Perkins, I. Simnett & L. Wright), 186–95. John Wiley and Sons Ltd, Chichester.

Illich, I. (1977) *Limits to Medicine*. Pelican, Harmondsworth.

Imperical Cancer Research Fund Oxcheck Study Group (1995) Effectiveness of health checks conducted by nurses in primary care: final results of the Oxcheck study. *British Medical Journal*, **310**, 1099–1104

Ingham, R. (1997) *When You're Young and In Love*. University of Southampton, Southampton.

Jonsen, A.R. (1998) *The Birth of Bioethics*. Oxford University Press, Oxford.

Katz, J., Perberdy, A. & Douglas, J. (2001) *Promoting Health: Knowledge and Practice*. Palgrave, London.

Kelly, M. (1996) *A Code of Ethics for Health Promotion*. Social Affairs Unit, Bury St. Edmunds.

Kennedy, I. (1983) *The Unmasking of Medicine*, 2nd edn. Granada, London.

Knowledge House (1992) *Better Living, Better Life*. Knowledge House, Henley-on-Thames.

Koehn, D. (1994) *The Ground of Professional Ethics*. Routledge, London.

Lacey, A.R. (1976) *A Dictionary of Philosophy*. Routledge and Kegan Paul, London.

Lalonde, M. (1974) *A New Perspective on the Health of Canadians*. Ministry of Supply and Services, Ottawa.

Lang, T. (2000) Cheap food, poor policy. *Times Higher Education Supplement*, 10 November, 19.

Lantz, G. (2000) Applied ethics: what kind of ethics and what kind of ethicist? *Journal of Applied Philosophy*, **17** (1), 21–8.

Lave, J. & Wenger, E. (1991) *Situated Learning: legitimate peripheral participation*. Cambridge University Press, Cambridge.

Lawrence, T. (1999) A stage-based approach to behaviour change. In: *Evidence-Based Health Promotion* (eds E. Perkins, I. Simnett & L. Wright), 64–75. John Wiley and Sons Ltd, Chichester.

McCormick, J. (1994) Health promotion: the ethical dimension. *The Lancet*, **344**, 390–91.

McCormick, J. & Skrabanek, P. (1988) Coronary heart disease is not preventable by population interventions. *The Lancet*, **338**, 839–41.

McGuire, C. (1992) *Pausing for Breath: A Review of No Smoking Day Research, 1984–1991*. Health Education Authority, London.

McKeown, T. (1976) *The Role of Medicine: Dream, Mirage or Nemesis*. Nuffield Provincial Hospitals Trust, London.

Marmot, M.G., Rose, G. & Shipley, M.J. *et al.* (1981) Alcohol and mortality: a U-shaped curve. *The Lancet*, 580–83.

Mill, J.S. (1962) *Utilitarianism* (ed. M. Warnock). Fontana, Glasgow.

Naidoo, J. & Wills, J. (1998) *Practising Health Promotion: Dilemmas and Challenges*. Bailliere Tindall, London.

Naidoo, J. & Wills, J. (2001) *Health Studies: An Introduction*. Palgrave, London.

National Pure Water Association (2001) *National Pure Water Association Web Site*. National Pure Water Association (http://www.npwa.freeserve.co.uk/) (20 June).

NHS Centre for Reviews & Dissemination (1998) *Smoking Cessation: What the Health Service Can Do*. NHS Centre for Reviews and Dissemination, University of York, York.

Nordenfelt, L. (1987) *On the Nature of Health*. D. Reidel, Dordrecht.

Nordenfelt, L. (1993a) Concepts of health and their consequences for health care. *Theoretical Medicine*, **14**, 277–85.

Nordenfelt, L. (1993b) On the nature and ethics of health promotion: an attempt at a systematic analysis. *Health Care Analysis*, **1**, 121–30.

Oxford University Press (1983) *The Oxford Paperback Dictionary*, 2nd edn. Compiled by Joyce M. Hawkins. Oxford University Press, Oxford.

Paton, H.J. (1948) *The Moral Law*. Hutchinson, London.

Perkins, E. (1999) Work with individuals – introduction. In: *Evidence-Based Health*

Promotion (eds E. Perkins, I. Simnett & L. Wright), 63. John Wiley and Sons Ltd, Chichester.

Perkins, E., Simnett, I. & Wright, L. (1999) *Evidence-Based Health Promotion*. John Wiley and Sons Ltd, Chichester.

Prochaska, J.O. & Diclemente, C.C. (1984) *The Transtheoretical Approach: Crossing Traditional Foundations of Change*. Don Jones/Irwin, Homewood, Illinois.

Pyne, R. (1995) The professional dimension. In: *Nursing Law and Ethics* (eds J. Tingle & A. Cribb), 36–58. Blackwell Scientific, Oxford.

RCGP (1986) *Alcohol: A Balanced View*. Royal College of General Practitioners, London.

RCP (1987) *The Medical Consequences of Alcohol Abuse: A Great and Growing Evil*. Royal College of Physicians, Tavistock Publications, London.

Reid, D.J., Killoran, A.J., McNeill, A.D. & Chambers, J.S. (1992) Choosing the most effective health promotion options for reducing a nation's smoking prevalence. *Tobacco Control*, **1**, 185–97.

Renaud, S. & De Lorgeril, M. (1992) Wine, alcohol, platelets and the French paradox for coronary heart disease. *The Lancet*, **339**, 1523–6.

Rodmell, S. & Watt, A. (1986) *The Politics of Health Education: Raising the Issues*. Routledge and Kegan Paul Ltd, London.

Rose, G. (1992) *The Strategy of Preventive Medicine*. Oxford Medical Publications, Oxford.

Russell, B. (1979) *A History of Western Philosophy*. Unwin Paperbacks, London.

Scadding, J.G. (1988) Health and disease: what can medicine do for philosophy? *Journal of Medical Ethics*, **14**, 118–24.

Scally, J.G. & Donaldson, L.J. (1998) Clinical governance and the drive for quality improvement in the new NHS in England. *British Medical Journal*, **317**, 61–5.

Scriven, A. & Orme, J. (2001) *Health Promotion: Professional Perspectives. 2nd edn*. Palgrave, London.

Scruton, R. (1986) *Sexual Desire: A Moral Philosophy of the Erotic*. Weidenfeld and Nicolson, London.

Secretary of State for Health (1992) *The Health of the Nation*. HMSO, London.

Secretary of State for Health (1999) *Saving Lives: Our Healthier Nation*. HMSO, London.

Seedhouse, D. (1988) *Ethics: The Heart of Health Care*. John Wiley and Sons Ltd, Chichester.

Seedhouse, D. (1995) 'Well-being': health promotion's red herring. *Health Promotion International*, **10** (1), 61–7.

Seedhouse, D. (1997) *Health Promotion: Philosophy, Prejudice and Practice*. John Wiley and Sons Ltd, Chichester.

Seedhouse, D. (2001) *Health: The Foundations for Achievement*, 2nd edn. John Wiley and Sons Ltd, Chichester.

Seedhouse, D. & Cribb, A. (1989) *Changing Ideas in Health Care*. John Wiley and Sons Ltd, Chichester.

SEU (1999) *Teenage Pregnancy: A Report by the Social Exclusion Unit*. Social Exclusion Unit. HMSO, London.

Skrabanek, P. (1990) Why is preventive medicine exempted from ethical constraints? *Journal of Medical Ethics*, **16**, 187–90.

Slote, M.A. (1983) *Goods and Virtues*. Clarendon Press, Oxford.

Society for Applied Philosophy (2000) Society information. *Journal of Applied Philosophy*, **17** (1), 127.

Society of Health Education and Health Promotion Specialists (SHEPS) (1991) *Register of Health Education and Health Promotion Specialists*. Society of Health Education and Health Promotion Specialists, Birmingham.

Society of Health Education and Health Promotion Specialists (SHEPS) (1997a) *A Career as a Health Promotion Specialist*. Society of Health Education and Health Promotion Specialists, Glasgow.

Society of Health Education and Health Promotion Specialists (SHEPS) (1997b) *Code of Professional Conduct for Health Education and Health Promotion Specialists*. Society of Health Education and Health Promotion Specialists, Glasgow.

Society of Health Education and Health Promotion Specialists (SHEPS) (1998) *Principles of Practice Briefing Papers*. Society of Health Education and Health Promotion Specialists, Glasgow.

Tones, K. (1983) Education and health promotion: new direction. *Journal of the Institute of Health Education*, **21** (4), 121–31.

Tones, K. (1990) Why theorise? Ideology in health education. *Health Education Journal*, **49** (1), 2–6.

Tones, K. (1992) Empowerment and the promotion of health. *Journal of the Institute of Health Education*, **30** (4), 133–7.

Tones, K. & Tilford, S. (1994) *Health Education: Effectiveness, Efficiency and Equity, 2nd edn*. Chapman and Hall, London.

United Kingdom Central Council for Nursing, Midwifery and Health Visiting (UKCC) (1992) *Code of Professional Conduct*. United Kingdom Central Council for Nursing, Midwifery and Health Visiting, London.

United Kingdom Central Council for Nursing, Midwifery and Health Visiting (UKCC) (1996) *Guidelines for Professional Practice*. United Kingdom Central Council for Nursing, Midwifery and Health Visiting, London.

Webb, D. (1999) Current approaches to gathering evidence. In: *Evidence-Based Health Promotion* (eds E. Perkins, I. Simnett & L. Wright), 34–46. John Wiley and Sons Ltd, Chichester.

Wikler, D.I. (1978) Persuasion and coercion for health: ethical issues in government efforts to change lifestyles. *Millbank Memorial Fund Quarterly/Health and Society*, **56** (3) 303–38.

World Health Organisation (1946) *Constitution*. World Health Organisation, New York.

World Health Organisation (1986) *Ottawa Charter for Health Promotion*. World Health Organisation, Geneva.

Yeo, M. (1993) Towards an ethic of empowerment for health promotion. *Health Promotion International*, **8** (3), 225–35.

Index

Note: Abbreviations used in the index are: CHD = coronary heart disease; SHEPS = Society of Health Education & Health Promotion Specialists; UKCC = United Kingdom Central Council for Nursing, Midwifery and Health Visiting